Life in the
Deadly World of Medicine

Joseph T. McFadden

This book is a work of fiction. Names, characters, places and incidents either are products of the author's imagination or used fictitiously. Any resemblance to actual events or locales or persons, living or dead, is entirely coincidental.
Copyright (c) 1999, 2002, 2007 Joseph T. McFadden

All rights reserved. Except in the case of brief quotations embodied in critical articles and reviews, no part of this book may be used or reproduced in any manner whatsoever without written permission of the publisher.
Angus Publishing, Vail, Colorado, originally published The Wafer in the United States of America in 2002, in conjunction with The National Writers Press, Aurora, Colorado.
Fragments of "The Force That Through the Green Fuse Drives the Flower" by Dylan Thomas, from THE POEMS OF DYLAN THOMAS, Copyright (c)1939 by New Directions Publishing Corp. Reprinted by permission of New Directions Publishing Corp.
Photo Chalice: O'Byrme Religious Goods, www.obyrneonline.com

Published in the United States of America
First Edition Hughes Henshaw Publications, August 2007
ISBN-10: 1439209553
ISBN-13: 9781439209554
eBook ISBN: 9781439290743
Library of Congress Cataloging-in-Publication Data
McFadden, Joseph T.
The Wafer / Joseph T. McFadden
p. cm.
1. Transplant 2. Donors 3. Cannibalism 4. Human Sacrifice 5. The Eucharist 6. Heart Surgeon 7. Courier 8. Wafer
Cover Design: Christina Estrada
Printed in the United States of America.

NOTE

Attempts to honor the *he/she* convention were found too cumbersome in the writing of this book, so the effort was dropped and the old style reinstated. The words *he* and *him* and *his*, as well as *she* and *her* and *hers* when used in reference to physicians, pharmacists, nurses, and others, mean anyone, without intended gender distinction.

This book should not be used to help plan a course of self-treatment. It is an advisory on avoiding mistreatment, mistakes, and accidents in the modern medical system.

TABLE OF CONTENTS

Chapter One:
MEDICAL MISHAPS   1

Chapter Two:
THE DOCTOR AND THE SCIENTIST   11

Chapter Three:
HOW WELL DO YOU KNOW
YOUR BODY?   23

Chapter Four:
ALTERNATIVE MEDICINE   39

Chapter Five:
IDENTITY AND CHILDREN   55

Chapter Six:
VIGILANCE, DOUBLE-CHECKING
RECORDS REPORTS   81

Chapter Seven:
DRUGS, ANESTHESIA, AND GASES   91

Chapter Eight:
BLOOD TRANSFUSIONS   121

Chapter Nine:
INFECTIONS   125

Chapter Ten:
X-RAY   145

Chapter Eleven:
PLASTIC SURGERY   153

Chapter Twelve:
A VIEW FROM INSIDE   157

Chapter Thirteen:
ERRORS, TRAPS, AND ACCIDENTS   165

Chapter Fourteen:
THE EMERGENCY ROOM   191

Chapter Fifteen:
THE BRAIN DEAD AND EUTHANASIA   195

Chapter Sixteen:
THE SITUATION   207

Web Sites   225

Bibliography   227

Chapter One
MEDICAL MISHAPS

Sick people and their concerned families turn for rescue to the world of medicine, the safest and most merciful of all human endeavors, so it would seem. But exposure to the system too often comes with another reality—the medical arena is no different from other human endeavors and in some ways can be worse, the astonished and grieving relatives left in a state of shocked disbelief, as happened to a lovely middle-aged lady, a devoted, concerned wife, Betsy Simmons. She arrived at City Hospital about 9 o'clock on a spring morning in a happy mood because her husband, John, would be discharged before noon if his improvement continued as expected. His recovery from a near-fatal infection had been almost a miracle, if not really a miracle, and she would be so happy and so thankful to have him home again. She felt good about the doctors and the hospital with its millions and millions of dollars worth of the most modern equipment: CAT scanners, MRI machines, the best of laboratories, highly trained staff specialists, and everything needed to be progressive in the modern world. The community was lucky indeed to have one of civilization's greatest blessings, a first-rate medical center and competent doctors. She intended to show her appreciation to each of them personally with little gifts and thank you notes as soon as she got John safely home.

She took the elevator to the fifth floor, stepped out into the hallway toward her husband's room, and waved as she went past the huddle of nurses poring over records in their glass enclosure. She tiptoed on down to her husband's room and slipped through the open door. At once a scream broke the silence of the ward, and Mrs. Simmons ran out into the corridor shouting, "Oh, my God! No! No! No! No!"

Nurses and other personnel rushed to the room and found John Simmons corpse-white without a pulse or signs of breathing, and lying terribly still in his blood-soaked sheets. Frantic resuscitation attempts produced no response, and no one in the room could deny the awful truth. Mr. Simmons had bled to death. He had been alone for at least two hours without anyone looking in on him.

Aghast and in a state of surprised shock, everyone asked the same question. What on earth could have happened to Mr. Simmons? He had recovered well enough to go home, and he had not been expected to die, even at his sickest. But his illness on admission required massive doses of antibiotics and large quantities of intravenous fluids. Frequent injections damaged and threatened to destroy the usable veins in his arms, so he had been given a subclavian line. Subclavian means under the clavicle, or collarbone. The line is a tube (catheter) sewn into a vein with its farthest end threaded down into the central venous system deep within the body. Doctors insert a central venous line when long-term treatment will be needed. Fluids containing drugs and nutrients are fed through it toward the heart, where it quickly crosses over into the arterial system to be distributed throughout the body.

Mr. Simmons had responded to the antibiotic treatment fed through his subclavian line, and the doctor had written an order the previous evening for the tube to be removed the following morning. Nurse N. came into his room before 7 a.m., tired from a night on duty, and harassed by having too much to do and too many patients to watch. She shut off the pump, disconnected the warning beeper, and had just grasped the lower end of the fluid line to remove it from the hub of the apparatus when a voice from the intercom shattered the morning hospital murmurs and demanded her immediate presence back at the nurses' station. The night supervisor, the authority to ordinary nurses, was in a hurry to go off duty, and something had made her very angry. This particular supervisor especially terrified Nurse N., who was a peaceful and somewhat whiffling innocent. Nurse N. flinched, releasing her grasp on the fluid line, and ran to the desk.

Half an hour later, Nurse N. went off duty crying, the victim of humiliating verbal abuse. The night supervisor had discovered an infraction in record keeping and blamed the young nurse for the problem. Meanwhile, Mr. Simmons wiggled restlessly, and the loosened tube end slipped out of its socket. He bled quietly from the open end of the line and lost consciousness. Mr. Simmons never called for help. He died at the most dangerous time of the day, when the night ends, and nurses change shifts. In this daily 7 a.m. ceremony, nurses who have been on duty all night turn over the patients to the crew arriving in the middle of heavy hallway traffic. The scene is edgy with an air of confusion. John Simmons died because no one had been watching him.

This incident caused no public reaction and elicited no response from law enforcement officers or from professional-conduct monitors. The news reached the local papers only as an obituary and drew no national attention. The victim, prominent neither politically nor otherwise, left no relatives except his stunned wife, who reacted only with defeat and caused no disturbance by attacking the hospital or suing her doctor.

Then the happening of this preventable death became an anticlimax in the silence of history because such quirks of fate are so unexpected. The infrequent news media reports of medical mishaps such as this one usually are ignored because the events seem remote from everyday reality. But within the past decade increasing evidence has stimulated concern and provoked statistical evaluations and other investigations into the world of modern medicine. As a consequence several recent studies claim altogether the astounding sum of 100,000 to 300,000 preventable deaths a year in the medical system of the United States. Reaction from the public and from patients and doctors alike to this disturbing news, as would be expected, has been disbelief. Impossible! Surely, these figures can't be right! And who says so, anyway? Hospitals are the safest of shelters, and doctors and nurses the most competent of keepers. Right? Besides, there is no other place to turn when illness strikes with the threat of death, a time when patients and their families want someone with knowledge and the ability to take over and get them out of trouble, someone to trust completely. In this mood people tend to surrender to the system; it's too complicated anyway for outsiders.

So, a closer look to see who is talking reveals facts even more sobering; the tabulations have been coming not from activists, sensation seekers, advocates of other therapies, or self-assured crazies, but from reliable and important sources such as the Institute of Medicine of the National Academy of Science, and the **New England Journal of Medicine** among others, and the reports continue. Now, on this foundation the news has a somber tone and a significance, indeed, of the utmost seriousness, the problem much bigger than anyone suspected.

Yet, as a practical matter, how could an accurate count be possible across the entire field of medicine with its thousands of doctors, its hundreds of hospitals in the system, the related gigantic drug industry, the insurance involvement? Overlap in the various tallies surely has to occur in so vast a territory, but whatever the final sum might ultimately prove to be, something really is amiss, the numbers entirely too big, very big indeed. Realistically, if the counts are anywhere near correct, it would be about six times more fatal to lie still for the medical establishment than to join the maniacs in traffic on American highways, where only about 50,000 are killed each year and several million injured.

Unless one of these medical tragedies has happened to a friend or a family member, a person might be quite skeptical. The unfortunate mishap of John Simmons is not recounted here to diminish the reputation of the modern medical system of the United States. In many ways it is the best the world has ever known, praiseworthy for its miraculous accomplishments. Attention to the flaws can only improve its services to humanity. But despite concerted efforts, no authority or organization has been able to eliminate the fatal faults. If the doctors, hospital industry, insurance industry, and the drug empires can't or won't control the damage, then who can? One choice remains. Only the patients and their families are left to confront the problem.

This calls for greater understanding of modern medicine, with its wonders and dangers, from earlier times to the present day. No one born since the end of World War II knows the grim limitations hampering medicine until well into the twentieth century. The introduction of sulfa drugs in the 1930s and penicillin in the early 1940s brought the first real defense against one of the greatest threats to life, infection caused by bacteria and other organisms. Since this beginning, the continuing advances in technology, in drug research, and in the understanding of disease processes have saved countless lives and cured countless people.

The doctor at best only prolongs life and delays death. He diminishes physical damage and alleviates suffering and anguish. His effectiveness continues to grow as medicine adapts discoveries from the scientific community to the struggle against disease. But slow as the progress of medicine has been over the centuries, the related social and economic issues have become by comparison a very damaging failure. The intrusion of government into the social and financial problems of medicine, the big-business tactics ruining the HMOs, the dictatorial control of medical decisions by the insurance companies, the drug industry tactics, all in the wake of revolutionary medical discoveries, have swept the doctor and his patients into a gigantic out-of-control industry where system failures are taking a terrible toll. Actually, these parts of the entire system meld to create a deadly void around the patient.

Under the current circumstances what can anyone do for himself or for a family member as a patient in this intimidating system? The answer is neither easy nor simple. Barriers have to be crossed, some ages old, and some almost forbidden by custom and tradition. A person would have to become an advocate and get involved, and expect to meet resistance. He would have to look for the weak places in the system. For instance, the handling of medication routines carries one of the major risks to patients. The responsibility for drug delivery as well as general administering to patients in a hospital and elsewhere is passed down from the doctor to people with less training. Each time a task changes hands, the potential for error increases. The doctor orders the medicine, and the nurse gives it by whatever route. The nurses' aides and maids do menial tasks like tending to bedpans and food trays, to free the nurses for more sensitive duties. Orderlies carry the patients by wheelchair and gurney to various places in the hospital. Each endeavor leaves room for error. Anyone exposed to this scenario soon comes to ask who is in charge of an unthinking person doing supportive tasks, and who is in charge of an unthinking person doing dangerous tasks? The answer becomes obvious, and it is not comforting. Quite simply, NO ONE IS IN CHARGE! No one is in charge because each employee is responsible for his or her own activity, with commitment to an assigned duty under a supervisor somewhere in the vicinity, but no one is in charge of the patient. So, this vacancy needs to be filled by the person who can see the most and do the most to safeguard any one patient, someone with an active mind at the bedside. And down to basics, only the advocate or the patient is the final guardian against mistakes where they are most likely to happen.

If the system is to be improved, the major offenders such as errors, accidents, drug misuse, infections, and human foibles, among other faults, must be brought under control. In the modern medical system as it continues to develop, the possibility of mishaps continues to increase, especially in areas where financial strictures are applied for the sake of profit. Patients caught up in these circumstances can no longer complacently regard the medical scene with the attitude, "It can't happen here." It does happen here, and patients and their families must learn to recognize the dangers and how to avoid them. In other words, it is time to empower the patient. And what would be the source of such power? Simply put, the answer is **knowledge**.

Here in an age of enlightenment, information available to anyone is also there for everyone, simply for the asking, from sources like Google, Wikipedia, etc. And it might help to continue an inside tour with the author who has been there, and over a long period of time saw the flaws and the weaknesses again and again. Every mishap described in this book is based on an actual occurrence; it really happened, the identities, of course, are disguised.

Chapter Two
THE DOCTOR AND THE SCIENTIST

The history of doctors and medical schools dates back to about 3000 B.C.; Imhotep, the earliest on record, came to be the god of medicine during the third dynasty of ancient Egypt. But the type existed far earlier in the development of humanity; drawings on the wall of a Pyrenean cave (about 15,000 B.C.) depict a medicine man at work. Actually, the original, the shaman, the witchdoctor, the same person by other names is probably as old as mankind, with his pain and suffering and fear of death. Hippocrates in fifth century B.C. became the Greek god of medicine, and Galen's teachings (second century A.D.) held sway for some 1,400 years, most of the prevention ideas right and his treatment ideas wrong. Not until the Flexner report of 1910 A.D. were the standards raised to a better and more uniform choosing of students and the adaptation of the latest in scientific progress to the practice of medicine. Throughout this long period very few regimens of treatment endured. In fact, most of them proved to be not only useless but also harmful, if not deadly.

Here in the early years of the twenty-first century the doctor (M.D.) must earn a high school diploma (four years), a bachelor of science or arts or a comparable degree (four years), and an M.D. degree (another four years). These years are followed by a period of postgraduate training, varying from a one-year internship to as much as 10 years in a surgical specialty. A plastic surgeon, for instance, who goes beyond cosmetic work and is trained to do major reconstruction, may be board-certified in general surgery (five years), in plastic surgery (three years), and a sub specialty such as hand surgery (one year). This adds up to nine years of training out of medical school and 17 years out of high school.

There can be no doubt about this doctor's significance and his commitment to excellence, his compassion and humanitarian impulses, or about his intelligence and unselfish dedication to caring for the ill. He never refuses to treat an indigent patient. He never refuses to teach medical students, nurses, or younger doctors in training. He is a gift to his community and his profession. There has never been anything like the modern medical doctor when he is the right stuff. He is capable of saving life in dozens of ways.

After training he becomes a part of a medical community somewhere, either on a medical school faculty with its medical school hospital, or as a member of one or more community hospital staffs. In either place, the doctor is not in charge. None of the hospital personnel work for him, and none are accountable to him. Doctors are not in charge of the hospital; administrators are, and they and the doctors often clash. In a hospital the doctor is dependent on the hospital's supply system for drugs and instruments and the personnel who work with him. So, obviously, much goes on here beyond his control.

On the other hand, the doctor might not quite measure up to this highly trained person; there are all grades below the really competent. And the hospital administrators have to suffer fools, too. Expensive and unproven new equipment demanded by inexperienced or unwise doctors may never prove be beneficial to the patients or profitable to the hospital. The situation calls for diplomacy and good judgment.

To whom is the new doctor in town responsible when he arrives to set up a practice? Actually, he works under no immediate authority except his own conscience as it guides him toward the reputation he seeks to establish. He does not have a boss. Will he tackle difficult and dangerous problems without previous experience or without consulting seasoned practitioners of his particular specialty? Do pride and ambition interfere with his caution? Are his failures called God's will, when someone else could have helped the patient? Doctors in well-known private clinics and in medical school hospitals with closed staffs have greater supervision, yet some of the very best doctors are outside in private practice. A patient has to get to know the landscape in order to find them.

The inertia of the hospital system tries to pull even the best down to its level. How well surgical patients do, aside from the surgeon's own operating room expertise, depends on how carefully the doctor rides herd on the staff taking care of the patients before and after surgery. But the doctor can't be everywhere at once. He has to go home for rest, and with critically ill patients in the hospital, his sleep might be fitful. The doctor might wake to call and check on the condition of someone and not be surprised to find an undetected disaster developing until the call prods the people on duty. This is certainly not a fail-safe method, and the doctor can't do this too many nights in a row without dropping from exhaustion.

So, how should a person go about protecting himself in this situation? First, the patient's choice of doctors is critical. There is a tremendous difference in talent and integrity among them, and the bad surgeon carries greater risk than the fellow armed only with pills and the like. Wise and experienced observers say, "The surgeon makes book on himself each time he operates." Choose wisely. There are certain dangers in today's HMOs. There the choice may be limited. In some organizations, the family doctor is actually compensated for not referring patients to a specialist. The patient in these circumstances may be forced to insist he needs or wants one.

How does a person find a good doctor, surgeon, internist, or whatever specialist might be needed? The answer to this question is not easy to come by, and its importance cannot be over estimated. The family doctor usually can be trusted to make the referral. Without this source or in a strange setting word of mouth can help. People who work in the hospitals know, but it is usually wise to get several opinions because personal likes and dislikes might color some of the recommendations. Among many other sources of information the computer has wrought a world of enlightenment and will continue to evolve as an almost limitless source. Start with the Yellow Pages for a name then go to an Internet search engine like Google and type in "American Medical Association" and click on "Doctor Finder." This source provides information on licensed physicians in the United States, some 690,000 entries, supplying basic information on the doctor's training. The AMA also publishes a four-volume **Directory of Physicians in the United States**, available in public libraries. Another source, **The Official ABMS Directory of Board-Certified Medical Specialists**, lists the names and the description of each person's training. This four-volume reference also can be found in public libraries. It lists all the specialists including family practices in each town, and provides a short biography describing the training of each doctor. Access to the ABMS directory can be had through a search engine, but some channels of information require registration and a fee. The reference books would serve better. Google can find a doctor if supplied with the name and location. Other sources include the Web sites of university medical centers. They provide basic information on the faculty members.

Information about any particular doctor can be found on one of several search engines. For instance, at **www.google.com**, "Virtual Hospital" is a digital library of health information. These routes reveal the training background of various specialists. HealthGrades, an online service, will supply a report on any physician for a fee (see their Web site at **www.healthgrades.com**). There is an ever-growing collection of information about physicians on various Web sights. Local people in a community know who is considered good and who is not.

A board-certified doctor has completed a course of postgraduate training in a chosen specialty and has passed an examination given by the board members of his particular field. The doctor has taken the training and learned the didactic material. The certificate means little more. It says nothing about manual skills, honesty, morals, dedication to excellence, sobriety, health, ethics, compassion, charity, or sanity.

Every state medical society maintains a Web site with information about its licensed medical practitioners. This includes a list of the physicians under investigation and those who have received disciplinary action.

If a diagnosis is not to your liking, other opinions are invaluable when properly obtained. Be wary of the method. The old adage "birds of a feather flock together" especially applies to medicine. It is safer to seek the second opinion independently. If the source of the first opinion makes the referral to the source of the second opinion, he is not likely to pick someone who is a threat to his own level of competence. Also, when one doctor asks another doctor for a mandatory second opinion on behalf of his patient, usually through a planned arrangement for such examinations, there is a tacit agreement against the second doctor's taking over the treatment, and a tendency for the two to agree. Go for another opinion instead of a second opinion, and without a referral from the source of the first opinion. This route makes it easier to choose another doctor. No one belongs to any doctor, nor does the doctor belong to any one patient until committed. Doctors make mistakes too, and misdiagnosis is not an infrequent occurrence.

Whatever characteristics are to be found in people in general will be found in doctors, too, from the near perfect, gifted, capable, dedicated humanitarian, to the callused crook and the murderous psychopath, and just as dangerous, the inept person who is blinded by his own egotism. With any new doctor be careful until you know.

THE SCIENTIST

The practitioner who is a doctor of medicine is not a scientist in the true sense of the word, and reminders of this fact infuriate those who pretend to be. If a doctor sees patients, he is a practitioner who uses his knowledge of medicine and the knowledge of other people in the world of medicine to direct the treatment of patients, and he does indeed apply many scientific principles simply because much of his information, plus the drugs, the technology, and most of the advances come from laboratories manned by researchers, some of whom really are scientists. True, controlled clinical trials have been used in the past, some leading to spectacular advances, and many more should be done in the correct manner; however, application at the clinical level is often haphazard; in numerous circumstances the practice of medicine does not lend itself readily to the rigid rules of scientific validity.

Striking examples are the treatment of infections and the use of drugs. Progress in both depends upon a background of continued laboratory research extended to the field of clinical use. Antibiotics given to patients who complain of a bad cold may stop a secondary infection. Under these circumstances the doctor will not wait for proof of such bacteria to be causing a progressive illness developing into sinusitis or bronchitis and pneumonia, or for the offending organism to be identified by laboratory studies. These can be fatal complications, and no doubt an antibiotic will sometimes beat a bad bug to the pass. According to accepted thinking it stops the development of pneumonia or other complications leading to death in an unknown number of cases. A modern example is the fourday packet of the generic antibiotic, azithromycin, for the patient whose bad cold has developed into sore throat, productive coughing, or slowly progressive worsening of disabling symptoms. The drug probably has a high hit rate. Antibiotics also get a lot of innocents along the way, including the internal flora necessary to normal life. Perhaps worse, this approach to treatment also contributes to the development of bacterial strains resistant to the known antibiotics, the price society pays for the blessings of the era. Yet the patient leaves the doctor's office reassured by the antibiotic and more than likely will not have to make another office visit for the same condition. The illness may or may not run the course it would have run without the antibiotic. Such treatment has a certain practicality, but it is not scientific. These remarks are not offered as criticism; they merely state the circumstances.

Medicine has always had its fads; today's knowledge might become tomorrow's ignorance. Harmful treatments worse than the diseases, one after another, have been used down through the centuries, and then abandoned as knowledge evolved. Among the common practices, bleeding (phlebotomy), harsh laxatives, and enemas as part of treatment further assaulted the patient's state of health by compounding the fluid depletion. Dr. Fagan, an eighteenth-century French court physician, became known as the "killer of princes." Louis XV survived a violent contagion at the age of 2 only because his nurse hid him from the purges, emetics, and potions prescribed by Fagan. All other members of the royal family died under his treatment.

Only in the early twentieth century did advances in the knowledge of fluid metabolism and physiology put a stop to these harmful practices. The new methods were devised to replace lost body fluids through the veins. Nutrient mixtures in a base of water and salt thus administered have saved the lives of thousands of dehydrated and depleted children and adults alike.

Progress in basic knowledge brought improved treatment and caused the abandonment of harsh and harmful treatments in many other medical problems. The outmoded prefrontal lobotomy is an example. It was first performed in a Swiss psychiatric hospital by Gottied Burckhurdt 1890. John Fulton at Yale University refined the operation and performed it on a primate, his monkey, Becky. In the 1930s Egas Moniz of the University of Lisbon's Neurological Institute proposed applying an improved version of the operation to treatment of certain mental problems. His colleague, a Portuguese neurosurgeon named Almeida Lima, did the surgery. For his contribution, Moniz shared the 1949 Nobel Prize for Physiology or Medicine with Hess. The operation made possible the management of out-of-control psychotics (obsessive hand washing until the flesh is worn down to bone, or fatal head battering against the walls of padded cells, and other unmanageable situations). Beginning with advent of the drug Thorazine in the early 1950s, the growth and development of psychopharmacology replaced the need for this irreversible and destructive surgery. The list of outdated treatments could continue, but the point has been made.

Concern over fallacies inherent in the concept of science as the only realm of fact has led to critical rethinking of its meaning and status in the human experience. Faulty thinking in the application of scientific principles to the evaluation of surgical procedures as well as to drug therapy has stimulated efforts to redirect assessment of treatment results. Medical statistician Major Greenwood, writing in 1923, regarded surgeons' handling of surgical statistics as comic opera performances. Today we have other guidelines for clinical practice such as those produced by the Cochran Collaboration. Its international electronic database is considered superior to the reports in medical journals. To obtain the evaluation of a particular treatment, Cochran Collaboration reports are available on the Web through search engines such as Google. Public libraries either have or can get this information. The Skeptic's Dictionary (**www.skepdic.com**) offers insightful evaluations of several misleading concepts.

Certain terms commonly used by scientists or would-be scientists create the air of validity. Among them **double-blind study** can be misused in conventional medicine to justify claims to the scientific method. Such claims stimulate peer respect and maybe envy. They support the pose to authority and under other circumstances try for credibility in endeavors such as certain alternative therapies, drug company claims, the pursuit of academic careers, and the competition for continued approval of grant money. The technique is open to question in many situations involving live patients, where too many variables are involved and too many causative factors for rigid scientific conclusions. **Statistically significant** is another frequently used term with the same implied claims of scientific proof, and its own set of results subject to interpretation. Both techniques are useful research tools when applied correctly.

The seriously ill patient with a condition for which a proven treatment otherwise is available should beware of becoming the victim of a double-blind study. Involvement in such a study should be only with the patient's full knowledge and consent. On the other hand, a person suffering from an unsolved medical problem might want to find an approved clinical trial where investigators are trying to apply scientific principles to the problems of treatment, while searching for a cure. See ***www.clinicaltrials.gov*** for more information.

So, what is the point? The answer lies within the nature of medicine itself. Nothing is black or white in all circumstances. The practice of medicine is both an art and a science, the term ***practice*** carrying a double meaning altogether too broad for hard science. Practice is another way of saying: ***keep trying until you get it right.*** The technology, therapeutics, techniques, knowledge, and understanding of diseases continue to change and evolve. The standard of excellence varies from door to door. Look in more than one place.

Chapter Three
HOW WELL DO YOU KNOW YOUR BODY?

The living body is a piece of machinery and like any other self-propelled vehicle requires an understanding of its works. Complicated though it is by comparison to the automobile, there are indeed similar maintenance problems and needs. She (the car) is getting older, maybe a little rusty around the edges, and has considerable mileage, but has served well, still runs beautifully, not anywhere near ready to quit. It is the same with the human body, but with much greater limitations. The body can't be traded in for a new one, and spare parts come the hard way indeed, if at all. This means greater care has to be taken with the original parts. And in doing so, it helps to know as much about the body as about the car, and to not take good health for granted.

THE NUMBERS

The simplest numbers—blood pressure, pulse, temperature, and the rate of breathing—vary on repeated counts, but their normal functions do stay within a certain range. Exercise, excitement, fright, anger, illness, injury, the weather, and many other conditions and events cause changes. Most people know the approximate number for each of these vital functions at rest: in adults 14 to 18 breaths per minute, pulse rate 60 to 100 beats per minute, blood pressure 120/80 (mm/Hg), and body temperature 97.8 to 99 degrees F.

Height and weight both change with age, and both will require a degree of remedial attention. Height-weight-age charts furnish a normal or average range, and body mass index (BMI) measures approximate body fat. All this information is available on Web sites including the method for calculating BMI, and several sites will calculate the figures.

BLOOD VALUES

Life depends on continuous complex chemistry of the body. Normal elements circulating in the bloodstream include fuel for the body chemistry, by-products of the processes, and structural parts of the blood itself, such as cells and fluids. Several dozen tests evaluate these properties, and under ordinary circumstances no one would be expected to have all of the tests performed or to know the results. However, a person in good health should be aware of certain baseline information about himself, such as blood type and the approximate numbers for red and white blood cells. As to the chemicals themselves, among the most important, the two cholesterols, the triglycerides, as well as blood sugar and electrolyte (especially sodium and potassium) levels, vary within a normal range. The baseline figures, along with the markers for cancer, infections, and heart disease, should be established early on in every patient's health record. For more information, log on to ***www.bloodbook.com.***

The circulatory system feeds and cleanses the multiple centers of this intricate body factory, and the average adult carries about 10 pints of blood traveling under high pressure at high speed, completing circulation from heart back to heart in about 30 seconds. Loss of a fifth of the normal blood volume means trouble, and the faster the loss, the worse the consequences if bleeding continues. Blood pressure drops, and the pulse races as hemorrhage leads to shock.

THE BRAIN

Several built-in mechanisms function continuously to protect the brain, which weighs 2 percent of the total body weight, yet uses 25 percent of the total body oxygen supply. Roughly a quart in size, it accommodates about a quart of blood passing through its vessels every minute. Consciousness depends upon this sustained flow bringing to the brain a life-sustaining constant supply of oxygen and glucose (a sugar). Unlike muscle and most other organs, it cannot store energy. If deprived of its blood flow for more than four minutes at normal body temperature, the brain will undergo irreversible damage. It uses many other nutrients, but not for basic energy, and the supply is not as sensitive.

The body maintains its own internal environment in a manner friendly to its survival. Many mechanisms designed to protect vital functions in changing conditions such as fright, flight, fight, pleasure, extreme weather, extreme danger, injury, bleeding, starvation, and exhaustion, come into action at a level below conscious will. These mechanisms depend on each other in their protective actions. When a person becomes exposed to extreme cold, the fingers and toes blanch or turn blue; the skin turns cold to the touch, and the pulse and respiration slow down, all in an effort to preserve core temperature. The brain, the heart and circulation, and the lungs must be preserved at all costs. Frostbite will claim extremities long before it nips the brain. In response to overheating, the skin flushes and sweats; the pulse and breathing rates rise to protect core temperature at a vital level.

The brain, the organ most sensitive to change, gets first claim on protection. When the carbon dioxide in blood rises 70 percent above its normal level, blood flow through the brain will double, and heart rate and blood pressure rise accordingly (Guyton, AC, Textbook of Physiology). This reaction serves to try to keep the brain's oxygen up to the required level. Increase the oxygen level, and brain blood flow decreases. If the brain were emptied of its blood, it would shrink more than 30 percent in size and collapse like a beached jellyfish. These facts may seem trivial to everyday existence, but they are not, because the brain is each person's universe. It controls who he is, and what he knows, does, and experiences. Hippocrates said as much more than two thousand years ago.

The cells doing the actual work of the brain, the neurons, number 100 billion to 200 billion. The cells supporting and feeding the neurons, the glia (glue), outnumber them by 10 to 50 times. Each neuron receives and sends messages to other neurons through multiple (1,000 to 10,000) connections called synapses. As many as one quadrillion of these connections serve the entire brain, the total length calculated to be between 100,000 kilometers to several hundred thousand miles. An accurate count is unlikely, but the number, obviously, is huge, and this anatomy creates the physical basis for some 100,000 chemical reactions per second in the brain to carry information across the synapses. These chemical agents are known as the neurotransmitters, and their study has created a burgeoning field of research predictably leading to greater understanding of human emotions and actions.

With its vast connections and control of endocrine secretions, the brain maintains a life-sustaining environment for its owner when it is exposed to threat. This happens without the person's having to think about the mechanisms set to come to his rescue. A surge of chemicals prepares the muscles for fight or flight and mobilizes the necessary energy. The vascular system constricts or dilates or both to deliver blood where it is needed and to protect the total volume. Numerous other reactions are stimulated by emergencies such as injury. The great physiologist, Claude Bernard (1865), called these phenomena "... the essential condition to a free life." Harvard physiologist Walter Cannon (1932) looked upon it as "the wisdom of the body" and gave its stabilizing effect on vital parameters a scientific name, **homeostasis**, Greek for **the same**. A wealth of detail about homeostasis can be found on Web sites.

DIET AND WEIGHT

Hucksters outnumber trained experts qualified to provide sensible answers about diet. Contrary to all the hype, most people simply need to find out what they are doing wrong and bring the bad habits to a halt. This approach will work better than the latest diet fads of high carbohydrate, low carbohydrate, low fat, high fat, or high protein, and other schemes. Awareness of a few basic facts will help in finding the right diet. Body energy comes from the breakdown of three fuel sources—carbohydrates, fats, and proteins—through a very complex system to produce a compound called adenosine triphosphate (ATP). ATP provides the energy source for all cells of the body, some 100 trillion of them. The simplest carbohydrate, glucose, provides the most immediate source of life-sustaining energy. The body has several mechanisms functioning constantly to keep the blood glucose level within normal range at all times because certain cells of the body survive only on glucose. These include brain cells (the neurons), red blood cells, cells of the retina, and cells of the gonads; only with glucose can they stay alive, and when the level falls below normal they are immediately in trouble. Furthermore, fats cannot be broken down except in the presence of glucose. If all carbohydrates were removed from any diet, body chemistry would break down protein and fat to provide glucose at safe levels for needed energy, and sugar would still be there. The body cannot sustain life without it.

The brain requires a constant supply of glucose. It uses 120g of the 160g needed by the whole body daily, and at any one time has only a two-minute reserve supply. The normal blood level of sugar varies from 70 mg/dl to 110 mg/dl. Hypoglycemia (blood sugar levels low enough to cause symptoms) begins below 70, with personality changes and altered behavior; a severe slow down signals a dip below 50. A glucose level dropping below 25 leads to convulsions, coma, and death.

The maintenance of good health requires a constant supply of carbohydrates in the diet. Complex carbohydrates are formed by sugar molecules of one type or another fastened together in chains, the links varying from two to several thousand, like the starches in grains, potatoes, and beans. The body breaks these down to glucose, and then burns the glucose for energy. Trouble comes from taking in too much of a highly refined sugar, mostly glucose. This single sugar molecule crosses rapidly from the gut into the bloodstream without the need for previous breakdown. This causes the pancreas to secrete a massive dose of insulin. The insulin too quickly causes this new glucose supply to be burned up, and the blood glucose plunges to low levels, creating restlessness, nervousness, hunger, even ill-tempered, out-of-control behavior. Cravings caused by this new low blood sugar level call for more food, which unfortunately, may be another fix of glucose. Because the starches and other complex sugars in fruits, vegetables, and whole grain products have to be broken down to simple sugars before combustion, a lower and more constant supply of glucose for energy can under normal circumstances be sustained from these foods without over-stimulating the secretion of insulin.

White table sugar is essentially glucose, the simplest and fastest-acting carbohydrate because it does not have to be broken down to a simpler structure before it can be turned into energy by the body. If the supply of glucose exceeds the immediate metabolic need, the excess is converted to glycogen and stored in muscle and liver for instant use when needed, and further excesses are converted to fat and stored. Excessive amounts of fats from food, as well as excessive proteins are converted and stored as fat.

Calories count. Glucose produces four calories per gram (15 calories per teaspoon of table sugar), protein four calories per gram, and fat nine calories per gram. Three thousand extra calories will increase body weight by one pound. And calories, apparently, are accumulative. To get a clearer understanding of the meaning of these numbers, consider a person who has a fixed caloric intake from established eating habits, and this includes one bottle of a sweet carbonated drink with lunch every day. Without changing anything else, stop the drink and substitute unsweetened tea or water in its place. The bottled drink has at least 100 calories, but usually more like 125 to 150. Working with the smallest number, this amounts to 3,000 fewer calories per month. On the new regimen, the person will effortlessly lose a pound a month, or 12 pounds in a year, and the weight will stay off. If the drink idea is not appealing, another niche in a person's diet might easily spare a hundred calories a day.

As sugar is abused and misused, so is salt. Watch people in a restaurant. very likely someone will pick up the salt shaker and dust his plate of food, including the salad, before he has tasted the first bite. The person who eats this meal takes on an unnecessary load of sodium, and sodium retains water in the body. Water weighs 8.3 pounds per gallon. The ankles, hands, eyelids, and belly swell, and he may gain five to 10 pounds overnight. Blood pressure goes up, and the heart has to work harder. If the person spares himself another overdose of salt, his body will begin to dump the excess water within a few hours, and weight loss may be rapid, like five pounds overnight. He will repeat the cycle until he learns to taste the food, not the salt.

Three sensible meals a day, or smaller amounts of food spaced more frequently, all containing carbohydrates, fats and proteins, will keep blood sugar within normal range in the well patient. By this mechanism the appetite will be subdued. In contrast, hunger defeats control. American society has the bad habit of trying to endure the long stretch from lunch to dinner without a break. The English custom of afternoon tea is like a much-needed fuel stop, and instead we have the cocktail hour somewhat later in the day. Americans arrive home exhausted, thirsty, ravenous, irritable, and have a drink. This means 300 to 500 calories before the meal. Within reach there might be a plate of crackers and cheese, or a bowl of over-salted nuts fried in unidentified oil. The treats are hard to resist, so conscience is eased with the deluding old excuse: ***they will absorb the alcohol.*** Then in the chase for sudden gratification the person reaches for a loaded cracker, and another, and another handful of nuts, until soon the calorie allowance has been used up, and dinner is not even ready.

Bad food, anger, worry, discipline problems with the children, lingering hostility over a problem at work, and other disturbances lead to overeating. So, what are some of the ways to curb the appetite? Good manners help. Eat slowly. The blood sugar level will rise, and the desire for food will diminish as it reaches normal range. The bad habit of eating too fast leads to overeating because the rapid intake of food outruns digestion. Bad food seems to stimulate a person to keep eating as though searching for something better. A food snob would walk off, which would be a good lesson for the cook. Calorie counting, certainly calorie awareness, at the table is a necessity to the control of weight. Don't eat the bread and butter unless they are needed for the count. A potato tastes good without the butter and high fat sour cream to disguise its natural flavors. Properly prepared potatoes and other vegetables such as broccoli, cauliflower, and green peas taste better without being doused in butter or another fat and salt. Their real taste may have been disguised for years, perhaps for a lifetime, until a person decides to try them in the barren state.

A pause for a few minutes at the end of a meal will allow the appetite to diminish as the digesting food does its work. When tempted by dessert, remember: If you eat it, you wear it. A single mint can stop the desire for a slice of cheesecake. Brushing teeth with a tingling peppermint toothpaste takes away the greasy taste lingering and diminishes the desire for something sweet after a meal. Watermelon fills quickly, tastes good to most people, is low in calories, and stops the impulse to eat something more damaging.

As to the mid-afternoon letdown—eat something. This snack should be an unrefined carbohydrate in a food source also containing fat and protein. Of the many available options, according to personal taste, a heaping teaspoonful of peanut (or another nut such as cashew or almond) butter is an excellent choice, but be sure to get real peanut butter (available at the grocery store) made from dry roasted or parched peanuts only, not the kind containing sugar and peanuts cooked in oil. The label has the facts. Raw, shelled peanuts roasted or parched to taste can be turned quickly to butter by a steel blade in your food processor. As another suggestion, try cheese without the crackers, raw fruit and raw vegetables, and unsweetened or lightly sweetened tea with lemon along with the food.

When shopping, read the labels and add up the calories. The differences can be astonishing. For instance, multigrain bread with 40 calories per slice is stacked on the same shelf with another brand containing 120 calories per slice. A quick energy bar with an athletic logo on its wrapper looks like a harmless healthy treat, but it may contain 250 to 400 calories. The load of simple sugar will goose the pancreas, producing a big rush, then cause further trouble in the fringes of hypoglycemia and out-of-control appetite. Any sealed wrapper with print on it should be read. The food inside has been processed and invariably contains one or more mysterious chemicals. God knows what they do to the body in the long haul.

Drinks containing alcohol are rich in calories and potent in stimulating the incautious appetite. Some sensible rules can help avoid trouble in the interest of both sobriety and weight control. First, never drink any alcoholic substance to relieve thirst. No amount will quench the desire for water because alcohol interferes with the normal glandular function inhibiting the loss of water through the kidneys, and therefore only adds to the water deficiency causing the thirst. The most overrated, a cold beer, does not relieve thirst. It does the opposite. Always quench thirst with water before starting on the wine, beer, whiskey or cocktails.

While the majority of fat problems may be due to unwise eating, there are numerous other causes which require medical investigation and professional management. The field of obesity has a long way to go in solving the problems related to variations in metabolism, those related to genetics, and to other causes.

BODY TEMPERATURE

Heating and air conditioning systems are about living within a viable temperature range. Too far in either direction can be fatal. Fifteen degrees Fahrenheit above or below normal is on the outer fringes. Over exposure to a hot climate can lead to heatstroke and dehydration (not enough body fluid), with body temperature of 106 F and higher (hyperthermia). This combination can be rapidly fatal and calls for emergency medical treatment. The opposite condition, hypothermia, begins at a body temperature of 96 F and becomes deadly below 90 F.

Surgeons and anesthesiologists deliberately use a state of hypothermia in some surgical procedures to protect the brain when its blood supply has to be stopped for a few minutes. The dangers severely limit the technique. At 84.2 F, heart irregularities begin to interfere, and below 78.9 F, the chances of cardiac arrest become too great. In a severe hypothermic state, a person can, from all appearances, be dead, with blue-splotched skin, dilated and fixed pupils, no immediately apparent pulse or blood pressure, and no reaction to stimulation, including pain. Some can be revived with the correct warming techniques.

Hypothermia occurs wherever the ambient temperature is lower than the body temperature. An old, poorly clad, debilitated person can die of this condition in a cold room at temperatures well above freezing.

Susceptibility to fatal exposure calls for protective clothing, shelter, and preventative measures. Eighty percent of body heat is lost through the head. Obviously, head coverage and other clothing is a must in cold weather. In the opposite direction, high heat and blazing sun are good reasons for wearing a cowboy hat.

MEDIC ALERT

A medical alert bracelet or necklace identifies preexisting conditions such as diabetes, epilepsy, emphysema, hypoglycemia, heart disease, cancer, allergies, and others. It's the first thing members of a rescue squad look for in an unconscious or severely injured patient. This jewelry identifies any abnormalities, the blood type, the nearest relative, the location of the medical record, and any variant from normal. The medical alert can help avoid mistakes and will speed up treatment. For the traveler, especially one with a known illness, this little tag might save a life.

Several organizations provide this service for a nominal fee. Among them, MedicAlert has been in operation since 1956. The Web site is ***www.medicalert.org***, or they can be contacted at MedicAlert Foundation International, 2323 Colorado Avenue, Turlock, CA 95382, (888 633-4298). Membership is $35 for the first year. MedicAlert on Google offers several other options for the same service.

Chapter Four
ALTERNATIVE MEDICINE

Alternative medicine includes all methods outside the limits of conventional modern approaches to diagnosis and treatment. Many people turn in this direction through impatience or desperation. The impatient use it out of frustration with doctors and the medical system, and are usually less likely to have a life-threatening condition. Desperate people turn to this source when conventional medicine cannot save them, and they are willing to try anything. Realistically, conventional medicine does not have all the answers and is still learning. It will continue evolving and incorporating new knowledge as long as there are patients. But we must not forget the facts about all human knowledge: it came from people struggling for answers through the ages, starting from a state of abysmal lack of usable information. Thus, the wonders of modern chemistry grew from a beginning in alchemy; our understanding of the universe with its mysteries of space and time and light started with the speculations of astrology, and many of our best and most reliable medical principles reach far back into folklore and folk medicine to a time ago when people fared as well on their own treatment as they did on the treatment available from medical practitioners. Many did better when they avoided certain harmful practices in vogue at the time, like the bleeding of seriously ill patients and commonplace use of harsh laxatives and depleting enemas as preventative measures against disease. Customarily and as a ritual at one time, most children received a spring cleaning-out with castor oil as a home remedy, followed by Epsom salt or other harsh laxatives, then enemas to finish the job. In the hands of the medical establishment, children and adults acutely ill from malaria, for instance, were cleaned out with a laxative and calomel before the first dose of quinine could be given, all for no good reason. Harmful treatments and toxic medications were used to the detriment of the ill by people in general and doctors themselves. Many if not most patients would have fared better without numerous accepted practices of the time.

Prominent among effective remedies coming from folklore and hearsay is the commonplace aspirin. Chinese healers used willow bark to treat pain in 500 BCE, and a hundred years later Hippocrates prescribed willow bark and leaves for pain relief. The effectiveness of willow was proven in 1753 AD. In the early twentieth century, laboratory studies revealed its mode of action. It contains salicin, which in the body converts to salicylic acid. Its descendant, the synthetic drug, aspirin (acetylsalicylic acid), was compounded in the late nineteenth century.

Another commonplace drug, quinine, came from Cinchona bark and has been in use for several centuries to treat malaria. For this purpose the growth of Cinchona trees is a major industry in several countries. The same bark contains quinidine, a drug used to treat abnormal heart rates.

The foxglove plant, prominent in folklore and myth, was mentioned in the thirteenth-century writings of Welsh physicians, and English physicians began using it more than 200 years ago in the treatment of heart irregularities and heart failure. It is the source of digitalis, known in medicine as a cardiac glycoside. Glycosides also came to medicine through the study of arrow tip poisons employed by various South American tribes. Strophanthus and squill, both sources of glycosides, were known to the ancient Egyptians, and were used in later times by the Romans to stimulate the heart. Toad venom and the dried skin of the common toad also contain glycosides.

These drugs and their derivatives are now very much a part of contemporary conventional medicine. A wealth of fascinating historic information on these and other drugs arising from folk medicine is available on various search engines. No doubt other therapeutic treasures and remedies are yet to be discovered in the forests and jungles and in the lore of folk remedies. Plant pharmacology begs for further research.

And there is the fascinating story of Edward Jenner, the English general practitioner who in the eighteenth century gave the world the modern smallpox vaccination. This discovery has saved literally millions of lives. Where did he get the idea? From a milk maid, when he heard her say she would never get smallpox because she had contacted cowpox from milking cows. Cowpox was seldom disfiguring or fatal, but it gave its victims immunity to the deadly smallpox, which killed untold numbers of people and left its few surviving victims terribly deformed.

HERBAL REMEDIES

Many herbs and teas have a medicinal effect, and some of the herbs currently in the ranks of alternative medicine will no doubt be assimilated into conventional medicine as evaluations continue. No intelligent person can quarrel with the use of herbs and other plants, but he certainly has legitimate reason to be reluctant about the foolish practice of using this approach to replace proven conventional medicine, and the indiscriminant and often deceptive mixing of both. Reckless claims for one or another herb should be received with skepticism.

To become a diehard adherent to alternative medicine and accept unfounded claims without doing adequate research is to join the ranks of the ignorant, superstitious, and foolhardy. Government regulation exerts a certain control over the use of drugs and treatments in conventional medicine, while alternative medicine, largely an unregulated industry, leaves the naïve and the gullible to fend for themselves.

Most ingredients in herbal remedies produce no recognizable signs of poisoning, but anything could be in the bottle just purchased. Since it is unregulated, the pills can contain something else, or be diluted to a useless level even if truly effective for any ailment at any strength. Herbal remedies may deprive a person of precious time when a treatable but progressive disease takes over. To act without the benefit of a doctor's guidance and knowledge is to keep company with the superstitious, who have done such things in the past as bathing newborns in stale urine and blaming illnesses on the work of the devil, sin, or divine justice. Some of the herbal and so called natural mixtures contain animal parts and animal excrement. Many adherents of alternative medicine are seldom bothered by doubt when taking unproven remedies.

Beware of positive statements about various herbs, weeds, and concoctions. For safety they should not be mixed with prescription drugs. Unless controlled studies have been done on a particular remedy, its effect on normal body functions—the everyday physiology and metabolism—is not known. In the body's complex chemical factory, a little of the wrong substance can be deadly. For example, a taste of cyanide or a drop of nicotine can be a fatal dose. Other natural remedies might have a more prolonged and subtle action, and a variety taken over time can have a cumulative effect, causing anything from minor illness to sudden death.

This is not the place to question or to support the claims for herbs such as ginseng, kava, Ginkgo biloba, St. John's wort, feverfew, or the many others. But it is the place to point out some of the dangers. The American

Association of Anesthesiologists warns against using interactive herbal remedies with conventional drugs and recommends the discontinuation of all herbal supplements at least two weeks before surgery. For instance, Ginkgo biloba increases the action of blood thinners such as Coumadin or aspirin, and may cause difficulty in controlling bleeding at the time of surgery and thus ruin an operation by postoperative bleeding. Kava accentuates sedatives including the action of alcohol. Ephedra (the Chinese *ma huang*) dangerously accentuates the action of stimulants, caffeine among them, and has been blamed for some deaths.

Before taking any herbal supplement resort to modern enlightenment. Get on a Web site and read about the remedies, the complications, the contraindications, but cull the hype put out by hucksters trying to sell the product. At this point something should be said about these people, something which no one should ever forget: they are in business to sell, and to do so they take reckless risk with human life and well being, and play loose and fancy free with the truth. A typical approach is to lead the person in need to believe the worst about doctors and medicine, accusing them and the system of hiding the truth for the sake of their own profit. Thus statements such as **what the doctors don't want you to know,** or **what the drug companies don't want you to know**, written or announced in such a way as to lead the person to believe there are miraculous cures for cancer and other deadly diseases being withheld or hidden in order to protect the doctors and the hospital incomes. At least one of these peddlers, an ex-convict, blatantly makes false statements with no evidence to prove his claims of deception by doctors and drug companies. He has made millions of dollars from his books full of misinformation and his at best useless concoctions. Anyone inclined to take such a person seriously should first go to the trouble of finding out the facts on one or more search engines such as Google. This also should be said—if a cure for a disease is available, the public here in the twenty-first century and the medical community will embrace it as soon as or even before it meets safety standards. Contrary to hiding effective treatment, they are desperately constantly looking for it. Their resistance to change wears down quickly in the face of successful treatment.

HOMEOPATHY

Samuel Christian Friedrich Hahnemann founded homeopathy in the early nineteenth century. To contrast his claims, he coined the term allopathy and applied it to conventional Western medicine. In this concept, allopathic medicine produces effects different (allos = opposite) from those of the disease under treatment, while homeopathic medicine mimics the symptoms of the disease. In truth, however, standard medicine does not honor the word allopathy as either a title or as a principle of accepted treatment. Both terms remain archaic in value.

According to Hahnemann, homeopathy helped the vital force in the body and restored harmony and balance.

These terms have no bona fide meaning when referring to specific body parts or functions. "Homeopathy" is the combination of the Greek words, homeo (similar) and pathos (suffering). Allegedly, homeopathic remedies come from minute quantities of minerals, herbs, and other materials. The remedies are diluted (from 1/10 to 1/1,000,000 and higher) with water or alcohol, or ground with milk and sugar, then further diluted and succussed (shaken). Shaking the extreme dilutions, Hahnermann claimed, made the substances more active and released spiritual powers. Many homeopathic remedies are available on the market. One of them, oscillococcinum (The Cochrane Library ISSN 1404-789X), is said to relieve cold and flu symptoms. Exhaustive testing has shown this solution of processed duck liver and heart to be diluted beyond any possible therapeutic concentration, if effective at any level.

NATUROPATHY

According to Naturopaths, the body knows how to repair itself and recover from an illness when provided with a proper healthy environment. Also, in their concepts, the natural body is joined to a supernatural soul and a non-physical mind, and the three must be treated together with remedies such as sunlight, air, and water, as well as diet and massage. Some of these concepts are, of course, entirely correct and the rest useless. The blame for many diseases, including cancer, falls on faults of what the

Naturopaths referred to then as the immune system (as it was conceived then), and they use vitamins, herbs, coffee enemas, colonic irrigation, and meditation to boost this system to fight diseases (Wikipedia.com).

Without doubt, exercise, a diet of fresh fruits and vegetables, and quitting smoking are healthy habits in any regimen of treatment or in just everyday living. Naturopathy becomes dangerous when used as a substitute for sound medical treatment of a recognizable and treatable disease.

Both Homeopathy (founded in the nineteenth century) and Naturopathy (founded early in the twentieth century) were superior to some of the treatments such as blood letting, harsh laxatives, enemas, and other harmful practices of conventional Western medicine at the time, simply by doing less harm. Both have declined sharply with the evolution of modern medicine.

OSTEOPATHY AND CHIROPRACTIC

The medical doctor (M.D.) and the doctor of osteopathy (D.O.) use the diagnostic and therapeutic techniques of conventional medicine. Thus indoctrinated, the D.O. in the USA is now allowed to train in the medical specialties and can obtain hospital privileges comparable to those of the M.D.

Other practitioners belong to the alternative medicine classification, among them chiropractors, who blame interference with nerve function for disease and profess to bring about a cure by adjusting the spine to relieve pressure and restore normal nerve action. They treat symptoms by performing a type of physiotherapy, and no matter what guise physiotherapy might have in the jargon of the practitioner, it is greatly underestimated in the aid it can bring to recovery from the aftermath of severely debilitating disease and injury, as well as to a host of unexplainable and unexplained aches and pains. But physiotherapy is not a diagnostic tool, and it is not used to treat diseases. It is used to treat the crippling aftermaths of diseases and injuries.

Why and how does the chiropractor get away with this slap in the face to conventional medicine? Quite simply, two things: talk with the laying on of hands, and the dismal list of failed and abandoned fads, some of them cruel, painful, and harmful, in medicine. In chiropractic the patient gets answers delivered in a positive manner, and the practitioner never bears bad news. He never has to tell a patient or family of impending death from an incurable disease. He puts the patient through no expensive, painful, or dangerous diagnostic procedures other than the money wasted and the unnecessary radiation exposure of the X-ray pictures and CAT scans, and the expense of MRI. He does not have to take a responsible approach to investigating the cause of the illness or the symptoms as defined by conventional medicine. He already knows the answer; the symptoms are due to interference with nerve function, which he claims to cure by manipulation of joints and the spine. There is no waiting for laboratory reports and no delay because of emergencies. The patient leaves the office with something positive: the practitioner has put his hands where it hurts. If conventional medicine were infallible, this situation could not exist. These practitioners are sustained and their coffers filled by the alternative medicine mentality. No life-threatening emergencies occur in their practice. Yet thousands of patients don't know the difference. Chiropractors carry the title doctor; they call themselves physicians, and the patients naively trust the title. If you are sick with a curable disease, you only delay treatment by taking this route.

Furthermore, physiotherapy of a harmless variety is available to you through your doctor, or even your private or public health club. Some physiotherapists are highly trained and highly skilled in rehabilitating the severely damaged patient, and work under the super vision of one or more medical doctors, usually an orthopedic or plastic surgeon from whom they get a steady flow of customers. Rehabilitation medicine has become a medical specialty itself and can help a patient work his way out of physical damage. It's better to spend money here than to be deceived by erroneous claims.

If the chiropractor does not cure diseases, can he do direct harm? Yes, he can and he has. Ill-advised manipulations and other violence to a patient's spine have led to tragedy. One complication from manipulating the neck of an old person with arthritic spurs on the spine is the damage done to arteries feeding the brain. This can cause sudden death or ruinous stroke. An abrupt maneuver jams a sharp arthritic spur into the artery or arteries, those encased in bony spine paths through the neck (the vertebral bones). Adjustments at this level of the body also can damage the spinal cord encased in arthritic bone, and the result may be paralysis from the level of injury down, maybe both arms, both legs, and all sphincters. Further down, manipulations to the back in the presence of a ruptured disc can and have caused paralysis of a greater or lesser degree, varying from a foot-drop to loss of control of the feet and the lower legs and sphincters of both bowel and bladder. Such patients need immediate correct diagnosis and emergency surgery to remove the offending disc material; otherwise, the damage will be permanent. Even then, total recovery might not occur.

Chiropractic has never saved a life unless it happened to prevent suicide with an exceptionally inspiring rubdown.

Medical school and a long course of postgraduate training is a tough route to go. Short cuts are an easy way to the money, a way to get there without being the real thing. Beware of the sign reading Doctor John Doe. Rest more assured with the sign, John Doe, M.D. The "Doctor" sign hides something: preacher, psychologist, Ph.D., chiropractor, social worker, a professor of something besides medicine, an outright fraud, and other possibilities, none of them the real thing. The article entitled, "A primer of complementary and alternative medicine commonly used by cancer patients," by Edzard Ernst(**www.mja.com.au/public/issues/174_02_150101/ernst/ernst.html**) presents controlled studies of acupuncture, diets, aromatherapy, chiropractic, herbal medicinal products, homoeopathy, and other methods. Web sites offer a world of information.

FAITH HEALING

Faith healing certainly has its place in alternative medicine. The term has to do with various sub-cults of organized religion and is used to claim miracle cures of terrible maladies such as blindness from the time of birth, deafness from the time of birth, paralysis, cerebral palsy, terminal cancer, pain, and even professes to have raised the dead. The method usually requires the laying on of hands. No records have been kept of its successes and failures. Skeptics of faith healing far outnumber its adherents. No one knows or understands the limits of this phenomenon, but whatever the power of faith healing may be, it carries a zero mortality rate unless it fatally delays conventional treatment of a progressive but curable disease.

Faith of a lesser sacred flair denotes trust in a system chosen by a person seeking help for his troubles, both mental and physical, and is often used as a means to an end. But everyone resorts to trust, regardless of the system, conventional or otherwise. Indeed, there is a certain amount of it in so-called scientific thinking. The entire spectrum of medical treatment, from the highest achievements in modern medicine to the unfounded claims of alternative medicine, is colored by remnants of the power and the mystery once wielded by the witch doctor. He had absolute power over the uninformed, especially those who could neither read nor write. The sick and frightened patient still sees some of this power in even the most highly trained physician.

The remedy in this confusing field lies, of course, in the realm of knowledge. Alternative and conventional medicine both get credit for cures due solely to the disease running its natural course without killing or crippling the patient. The medicine might or might not have had any effect on the disease, nor did it kill the patient. Internet search engines supply a rich source of information on alternate remedies including herbs, prescription drugs, and over-the-counter medicines.

Many books have been written on the subject of alternative medicine. Some dealing with enterprises contradictory to conventional medicine employ uncritical language, lending them a false certainty and a false sense of credibility.

There is no safe approach to alternative medicine. Taking herbs recommended by friends, none of them medically trained, is like swallowing strange pills out of an unlabeled bottle. With luck, nothing fatal happens. A healthy skepticism helps.

THEORY OF DISEASE

People throughout the ages have struggled to understand the cause of diseases. The theories in vogue now are of relatively recent origin in the scheme of history. Only in the latter half of the nineteenth century did infection by micro organisms come to be recognized as a major cause of illnesses. The idea still meets resistance from certain quarters. Other categories include the degenerative diseases, the immune system failures and faults, aging and deterioration of blood vessels leading to heart attack and stroke, abnormal cell growth as the central process of cancer, genomic aberrations, dietary deficiencies, and poisons to name only the more common causes.

Homeopathy, naturopathy, chiropractic, faith healing and others started on the basis of a theory of disease, all of them, as most people have come to know, more or less wrong. They thrived and gained power from the failures and faults of conventional medicine. While none of these endeavors ever provided a specific cure for a real disease, they at the same time, with one exception, did not make the patient's condition worse with harsh treatments, and never bore bad news. With the continued progress of medicine, these aberrations very likely will cease to exist.

Chapter Five
IDENTITY AND CHILDREN

The social standing of a patient, his age, the reputation of his doctor, and the nature of the disease will influence the attitude taken toward him upon his arrival at the hospital, and all these together will help determine his fate. The VIP, like the major contributor to the hospital building fund, or the President of the United States, will get a reception and attention not likely to be shown the person in a charity bed. A person of no particular distinction or one who shows no signs of inquisitive intelligence, is less of a threat to the hospital staff and can very easily become dismissed as a disease or a condition such as **the terminal breast cancer, the heart attack, the brain tumor, the thyroid, the lung cancer,** and **the pneumonia.** The formal name becomes secondary, the identity solely in a chart or a computer terminal at the nurses' station.

Here is an example. The restless, agitated patient, referred to as **the dental**, a nuisance in bed 16 of the recovery room, created a disturbance all night long. The nurses placed restraints on his wrists after the third dose of painkiller and two shots of sedatives, and he still wouldn't settle down. As daylight approached he really began getting seriously out of hand. He wrestled frantically and tore the skin on both wrists while trying desperately to get his hands loose. The nurse had the orderly tighten the cuffs three times. These stiff leather straps, a quarter-inch thick and two inches wide, in no way would yield to his efforts to tear out of them. The nurse called her supervisor and received an okay to repeat the sedation. But the annoying patient still did not stop the struggle, and no one on duty took him with real seriousness. He was just a dental problem. A dentist had extracted all the patient's teeth the previous morning under general anesthesia with a tube down the windpipe (trachea). The dentist had trouble with bleeding, and the anesthesiologist decided to leave the tube in place for safety against the patient's choking on blood oozing from the diseased gums. Dentistry is no big deal, anyway; dentists seldom bring patients into the hospital, and when they do someone else has to bear the responsibility for real medical problems, the anesthesiologist for the anesthesia, but who, then for other problems and complications? In truth, such a person too often has not been designated. And the thinking too easily can slip into this emotional vein—nothing significant could be wrong with this particular nuisance, nasty old rotten-toothed, stinking, sorry piece of humanity, repelling anyone who came close. As morning light crept into the room, the patient became wilder and more violent. His eyes rolled about madly and after awhile took on a desperate look.

At about 7 a.m. the patient's eyes began to bulge. He turned an angry, dusky color and made one final effort to free his hands, then suddenly stopped moving and went slack. A nurses' aide called out, and the nurse in charge hailed an anesthesiologist passing through the unit on his way to the operating room. He rushed over and tried to resuscitate the patient. Air couldn't be forced through the tube so he removed it from the windpipe and found it totally closed with junk and clotted blood. But the heart had stopped, and all measures failed to start it again. The patient had smothered to death, despite having fought valiantly to save himself. Had his hands reached the tube, he would have pulled it out and breathed.

This deadly situation developed in a modern, wellequipped hospital and grew to fatal proportions from an attitude. The person's illness, his physician (just a dentist), the nasty mouth, his noisy behavior, all relegated him to lesser importance, hardly more than a nuisance. The night nurse became determined to conquer his noisy fight. She would stop his unreasonable activity. He was bothering people; he was an enemy to the night; he was an inconvenience. The patient couldn't say a word around the tube down his throat. He could only grunt and sling his head, giving himself the appearance of a wild animal out of control. In her attitude, the nurse was blind to his animal-like and desperate efforts to communicate. The orders written on the chart, "suction tube PRN," went unheeded. PRN stands for **pro re na'ta** (according as circumstances require), which means **as needed**, and leaves something to the judgment of the nurse in charge. Her judgment proved to be poor, indeed, and what can be said about her behavior—uncaring, arrogant, and callused? Right! Yet she also has many good qualities. She is a nurse, so we know something commendable motivated her to study and work toward this goal. Ordinarily, she does her job with passable compassion, but something blinded her on this fatal night. She made a terrible mistake and will never be able to correct it because the patient is dead, and dead is forever. A vigilant relative, a friend, a sensible person by the bedside would have intervened and saved him.

Not too long ago, hospital personnel and physicians alike resisted the presence of a patient's relatives on the scene. Relatives and friends contaminated the rarified air of the inner sanctum. They brought in germs. They got in the way, asked too many questions, wasted the doctor's and nurse's time, and the restraints imposed by the presence of outsiders interfered with the freedom to behave as they pleased. The visitors might see something they're not supposed to see. Limited visiting hours were strictly enforced.

Those were simpler days. Now, the sensible doctor has come to respect and even depend on the presence of family members for help. A family can provide bedside vigilance if nothing else. No one would fall out of bed in the presence of an attentive family member, or tear open his surgical wound, or injure himself trying to get to the bathroom, or go unfed because he can't find his own mouth with a spoon. But, of course, some families could not be trusted with this responsibility.

No one is exempt from the dangers of mistakes and neglect and especially from faults due directly to reckless arrogance of the system. For this reason, identity should remain all-important to a patient during a hospital stay. Dignity, privacy, and formality are defenses against the everyday irritations of rubbing up against other people and events. These attributes give a person self-control in the presence of those with whom he interacts. They are not weapons so much as civilized ways of showing respect for self and for others. To really get to a person, one or more of these defenses has to be penetrated and put out of commission to weaken identity. Something has to be done to render the person powerless in the circumstances.

Depersonalization begins the moment a patient arrives at a doctor's office. Almost invariably a repressive attitude hangs in the air, no matter how polite, and something like the following scene unfolds. The receptionist might be very cordial and polite between telephone interruptions, but she might also give arrivals a greeting worthy of an intruder. Let's say an old retired surgeon, well known in the community, everybody knows Dr. John Smith, answers her query, friendly or otherwise, with, "I'm Dr. John Smith. I have an appointment with Dr. Gordon at 1 o'clock." Within the next minute, more often than not behind a smile, she will call him **Mister** Smith or just plain John. Respect and formality and plain good manners are of no consequence to her.

Then, no matter how many have been filled out in the past, more forms will be presented, once again, the name and address and phone number and the names of the medicines being used. There are dozens of questions to answer and yes-and-no boxes to check off. John Smith tells her none of this has changed, and she puts him down with the extremely wise remark about their wanting to keep all their data up to date, delivered in a tone of voice calculated to expose his lack of reason, then up pops the privacy form for signature. Of course, some of this is due to government intervention and interference, causing everyone to overreact to stay out of trouble. After this and other irritations, John takes a seat in the waiting room. The place is crowded, and no one is happy. Every patient has an irritating wait of undetermined length until called back into the hidden rooms. A surge of discouragement sweeps over him, and he feels an impulse to call the whole thing off, but he is there because he has to be. He is sick or thinks he might be, or he is there for a checkup to catch anything sneaking up on his state of health. He has come to take a chance on preventing the consequences of greater illness. So he gives in, and as soon as he surrenders, he will be moved about in a manner convenient for the system. From experience, he knew as much before he made the appointment.

John takes a seat and reaches for a magazine. Usually they are several months old and dog-eared, frayed, dirty, slick, and invariably ordinary. He goes through several before something catches his interest. Then in concentration he hears a familiar name being called out across the waiting room. His full name is John Robert Smith, and everyone on a first-name basis calls him Bob. He always introduces himself as Bob Smith. He hears this sharp voice calling, "John, John, John!" He looks up. The person, dressed in medical casuals and holding an armful of untidy charts, is looking at him, defiant. Again she yaps, "John!" He finally says, "Who are you calling?" She says, "John Robert Smith." Instantly, he wonders how they got on a first-name basis. What happened to his well-earned title, doctor, or the just plain dignity of mister? Why couldn't she cross the room and speak to him quietly? His impulse is to call her on her impertinence, but she would fill the doctor's ear after hours with her side of the story, and he does not want to stoop to anything small or petty. A person has got to be big under the circumstances. But he is uneasy and uncomfortable because of the humiliation in the waiting room full of patients. Old doctor, old farmer, old lawyer, old anybody, has been brought down to ground zero in the eyes of the crowd of common sufferers. Anyway, she is doing things the way they do things, the system in action.

As he is led into the next compartment of the office complex and toward the ultimate inner sanctum, his self-esteem suffers, his defenses against the system already weakened. Does the doctor really know what goes on in his own waiting room? Dr. Smith would bet not, and as he desperately realizes, he is in no position to tell his friend, the doctor.

The appointment progresses through a number of people before the doctor appears on the scene. Someone takes a history, and someone else checks height and weight, usually with clothes and shoes on and pockets full of keys and coins and wallets and pens and glasses; someone else checks the blood pressure through a layer or two of clothes, and another person does a partial examination. This casual attention to accuracy, to say the least, diminishes trust. Then the next wait in a small stall with his medical record flopped in a slot in the door and nothing in the room to read except the pictures of bisected human bodies or naked organs on the walls, gives a person time to think and reason and resent.

After awhile, the real doctor comes down the line. He picks up each record and enters one cubicle after another, taking the patients in serial fashion, behind schedule and with only so much time allotted to each. Through the walls, Dr. Smith hears the muffled sound of his progress. Upon entering a cubicle and confronting another patient, the doctor puts up a good front, the face of affable good humor, but down deep he's no happier to see the patient than the patient is to see him, under the circumstances. They may be cordial to each other or even friends out in the world, but here a problem must be dealt with, and he will perform his act to do it. If he were a lumberman, the next patient would be just another log to roll.

The patient, John Smith or otherwise, hesitates, and the list of symptoms in his hands remains unopened. He knows or has heard about the neurotics and hypochondriacs who take up a doctor's time needlessly with lists of numerous unexplainable symptoms to be explained, and he understands a doctor's dislike of lists, or thinks he does, and the disdain for such patients. Squirrels, the profession calls them. He would not want to fall into this category with his doctor, never again to get his real attention. So he misses his chance and says nothing while the doctor looks over the record, asks more questions, does some more examination, and is through. The patient shakes his head a little dizzily with a sigh of relief because he has come through the mill unscathed and has received no bad news. He is safe, once again in the clear.

Now wait. Smith knows this trap. Don't for one minute think the doctor can be comprehensive on every visit. Thoroughness is up to the patient. Has the doctor been told everything? Does the patient understand what he needs to understand before he returns home? If new symptoms have appeared since the last visit, a list will help. Otherwise, the patient will forget, or unconsciously dismiss the significance of his own symptoms. The physician is too busy to sort through all possibilities on repeated visits, and he can't really read another person's mind. Only the patient is responsible for his own body and his own health. The doctor is there to help, and he needs clues. But Smith has no new symptoms, so he lets it pass.

When finished, the doctor hands John Smith a sheet of pink paper on which he has made a series of check marks.

The receptionist who greeted him upon arrival takes the sheet of paper, looks at it, attaches another sheet with a stapler and addresses him, "All right, John, take this down to the lab, and they will do your lab work." There, before another receptionist, he might fill out more forms and sometimes repeat the same ritual when he reaches the X-ray department. The patient, Dr. Smith, begins to wonder. Do they lose what the patients are asked to fill out every six months? Do they put the paper to good use or just waste it? Don't they communicate with each other? Oh yes, the insurance cards, the receptionist has copied them every six months using the same excuse, they want to have the latest information on you. Does this treatment stimulate trust in the system? John Smith shakes his head and worries about his doctor for whom he has solid respect but nevertheless, he feels the sensation of slippery sands. After due thought he begins to understand. The system runs the doctors; they do not run it. The system works to reduce each patient to a manageable entity, to meet government regulations, and to compensate for irresponsible actions of patients at large. Some of the excessive work amounts to overkill.

We are talking about control. Control of what? Beyond the control of any one interest or group of people such as physicians themselves, money drives the system, whatever the endeavor. This does not necessarily imply greed on the doctors' part, but they all have to get through the day, pay the rent, pay for supplies, pay the office help, and the office help can work only so many hours. And time is out of control on the medical scene more than in any other place known to man short of war and natural disasters. Emergencies and the unexpected abound. The doctor who can completely control his time is not likely to be a very busy one, and if he is not very busy he probably is not very good at what he does, and people have caught on. Or he is in a specialty seldom visited by emergencies. Dermatology comes to mind.

To the matter of time, abuses do occur. As an example, let's say John Smith has become a chronic patient as he has progressed through old age. Osteoporosis has begun introducing itself, and he has fallen into the hands of a super-specialist who deals in the confusing field of endocrinology, or how the glands work and what to do and what not to do to appease them. Too little treatment and he will continue to shrink and shrivel, while on the other hand, treatment with hormones may cause or stimulate cancer growth, according to current thinking. So he needs careful medical monitoring in this sensitive situation, and he needs help with arguments for and against supplements. He drops the work of supervising the remodeling of his house, drives a hundred miles for an 8 o'clock appointment, and carries the 24-hour collection of his own urine into the spectacular clinic building of a famous place, and is welcomed by an unwelcoming attitude on two floors. The specimen should have been left at the laboratory. He received no such instructions, and no laboratory signs were found anywhere in the lobby. Subdued, he goes back the way he came and finally finds the laboratory out of sight around a corner on the first floor and gets rid of the jug without spilling a drop, then walks back upstairs to the reception area. Did he register downstairs? No, because the doctor is up here. He must register there first.

So, he goes down again, writes his name in a ledger; nothing else happens, and he returns to the waiting area upstairs and signs in there as well for his 8 o'clock appointment. By now it is exactly 8 o'clock, and a good thing he arrived 15 minutes early. Or was it? He is told to take a seat, and one hour later he is called in to see the doctor. During the conversation he tells the doctor he has stopped taking one of his prescribed medications because his stomach reacted violently. So, the doctor arranges for John Smith to get the medicine intravenously, and it has to drip in slowly over a period of three hours. Smith returns to the waiting room, where he sits for an hour watching people arriving and being called into the lab almost immediately. Then he is called in. The technician inserts an indwelling catheter into a vein, draws the blood samples, applies a dressing, and sends him through a different door to another receptionist, who takes the pink slip and tells him to have a seat. They will order the medicine, and it will take pharmacy an hour to prepare and deliver the dose. By then Smith has had enough, an hour's wait since the doctor ordered the medication, and now another hour's wait for it to be prepared. Why did they not obtain it during the first wait? "We can't until you bring this slip from the laboratory after your blood has been drawn." Why? he demands to know. "Because it's the way they do it," she says.

He abandons caution. He already has had a nasty encounter with the lab technician, who used un-sterile technique when puncturing his vein. He demands to see an administrator from the business office of this renowned institution. One hour and 15 minutes later, just after the drip has been started and John Smith is lying flat on his back, a young administrator arrives, stands over the supine victim and listens to John Smith's complaints about the unfriendly reception, the un-sterile technique, the long waits, and the attitude in general. The administrator is diplomatic and totally unyielding, and remains in the stance of standing above and talking down. Sterile technique, it has been determined, he explains, is not necessary in the puncturing of veins, and the clinic no longer requires it. Immediately, Smith feels as though his entire effort to be modern and keep abreast of things has been wasted on nonsense, and it has taken the astuteness of the business world to set him straight.

He started with an 8 o'clock appointment, waited an hour before seeing the doctor for less than 15 minutes, took another five hours to have a three-hour IV dose, and emerged from the clinic at mid-afternoon, feeling weak from hunger, diminished, depressed, and smoldering, but he can't do a thing about it. This doctor is the only endocrinologist in a city of half a million people and a surrounding population of more than another million, and Smith waited five months for his first appointment. Does he want to go to another big city and start over? No. He will have to put up with the system until enough people raise objections. The set-up functions to save the doctor's time and has no respect or consideration for the patient's time. Why is this situation more the rule than the exception? This doctor has no emergencies, and very likely he does not realize what is going on in his own office suite. The nurses and other personnel line up the patients, and he goes from one to the next. The sign-in log showed the names of several people who had 8 o'clock appointments with this same doctor. The patients have been grouped to avoid loss of the doctor's time, not the patients'.

In truth, the doctor is not running his own enterprise, and his underlings do as they please at the patient's inconvenience. There is another aspect. By habit of thought and tradition every doctor is a missionary in the foreign land of death and disease. He and his nurse make the team, and she leads him from one patient to the next, like Albert Schweitzer in the jungle. The destitute, the ill, and the frightened should be grateful for his presence. Only God could do better, and there is nothing in between. This team functions with a certain charity-ward demeanor, and regrettably, deceives the doctor, even in a high-end clinic. As put by an ethics professor at a southern university, "the doctor comes with a pedestal, and that's just the way it is."

To see the other side of the coin, travel down the road a few miles to a town of about 10,000 people and stop in for a visit at the family practice clinic. Pickup trucks jam the lot full, and the waiting area has standing room only, the chairs loaded with the obviously ill. These people don't bother with this place unless they are in trouble. It's first-come, first-served, no appointments. Five employees rush about in a clutter of records. No time is wasted here. The phone rings as soon as the receiver goes down, and the receptionist tells another caller, "Come on in, he'll see you, but it'll be at least an hour wait." The room is a descendent of the old charity clinics and charity emergency rooms, the training grounds of young doctors, where they learn their habits and their attitudes. Illness, disease, injuries, and death have no schedule. The doctor will get to you when he can. The last thing this clinic needs is another patient, and the one who leaves in a huff won't be missed.

MISPLACED TAGS

Identity by the tag method can be as simple as a band around a wrist or an ankle. Mistakes can lead to death, disfiguration, and ruined lives. Tales of the deliberate or accidental swapping of tags on newborns in the nursery are legion. Did someone accidentally do the swap before they were applied, or deliberately swap later to get a better-looking baby or to get rid of one with major health problems? Stories are legion and all too real about families who take home a child suffering from cerebral palsy or another devastating birth defect. They spend a fortune on treatment only to find out years later the tragic truth. The child is not theirs, and their own brilliant child has been in the wrong hands, deprived in the environment of a family of a different sort altogether. Imagine the bitterness and the frustration, the conflict of emotions, the sympathy and love for the child mistakenly given to them, and the outrage and anger at the people who put this family's own child into the wrong hands and deprived it of a rightful legacy.

Such mistakes can be avoided, and the means are at hand to correct them before a child is discharged from the nursery. As a last resort, DNA-matching tests on the children and the mothers can settle any disputes about identity. But parents should look carefully and without emotion. Is the child theirs? Does the child resemble them and other relatives? Any questions should be raised before the babies are released.

Misplaced tags can lead to another type of disaster, like this one in a big city hospital. Two short, obese, dark-haired men, age mid-40s, entered the emergency room minutes apart, each with a massive heart attack. They both died soon after arrival, and neither had an accompanying relative or friend. The family of one man came the same night and made arrangements with the undertaker to pick up the body for cremation. A relative of the second patient came the next day, a forlorn wife from another city. Her husband had been on a business trip when stricken. The body she was asked to identify was not the body of her husband. The tags somehow had been switched, and her husband had been carried out by the undertaker and cremated.

Who's to blame and how could it have been avoided? A hospital mistake was made, but the blame for the accident ultimately rests on an irresponsible relative who did not look carefully enough. Surely a concerned family member would have seen the body for correct identity before cremation. Possessions removed from the two men left no question about the identities. Without doubt the husband of the forlorn wife had been there; the hospital had his clothes and wallet and credit cards and driver's license. The misbegotten ashes of cremation were hers to keep.

THE WRONG PATIENT

Incorrect identity within the hospital can lead to disasters, and the possibilities are almost endless. The first among these is the wrong patient. This mistake seems to happen most often in pediatrics. **The pneumonia** was sent to the operating room to have his tonsils taken out. Such mistakes could be avoided by involving the parents or guardian in the hospital maneuvers. The parent or guardian might go along when someone appears with a gurney or wheelchair to roll the child to the laboratory, X-ray department, physiotherapy area, or the operating theatre, then upon arrival, stay with the child until hospital personnel claim the patient. Double-check identities, diagnoses, and intended treatment, and be especially vigilant if the trip is to the operating room.

While on the subject of surgery, here are other possibilities involving identity. The scenario goes like this. While the surgeon scrubs his hands and arms out at a hallway sink, the anesthesiologist puts his patient to sleep in an adjacent room. The operating crew swabs the skin at the site of the operation with a sterilizing solution such as Betadine, and then covers the patient in drapes for surgery. Nurses of varied experience do this, or young doctors in training, they too of varied experience. When the surgeon enters the room he sees the hanging bottles of fluid, the tent shape of drapes, but he does not see much, if any, of his patient. The patient actually might be face down for certain operations and, of course, not readily identifiable. In the patient's supine position, the face may be difficult to identify with certainty, distorted as often happens with a tube in the mouth and tape stuck to the skin, and the eye covers on. In these circumstances it is easy for a patient's identity to be mistaken. Who is under anesthesia and hidden in the drapes? Almost a hundred percent of the time, it is the right patient, but not always. How does this happen? The production-line mentality of the hospital, the collective mentality of the operating room personnel, or even the mentality of the surgeon, all contribute to the error. Unless he has well-trained senior residents and assistants to do the same for him, the surgeon himself should see each of his patients and look over the chart in the operating room, and speak to the patient about the operation before the anesthesia has been started.

In addition to getting the right patient, the correct area of the body should bear the operation. A good arm or leg too often has been taken off, leaving the bad one, the one intended for the amputation. The wrong kidney has been removed, leaving the bad one, the wrong side of the head opened, the wrong side of the chest. If the patient has two of anything, the surgeon and operating room personnel should double-check for correct orientation. What can the patient do to prevent such errors?

Either the patient or a relative can use a felt pen and write, "Don't remove this one," on the good arm or leg, or "Wrong side" on the normal flank skin, or "Bad kidney," on the bad flank, and show the art work to the doctor. And don't try any pranks like deliberately switching sides. Have a relative accompany the stretcher to the waiting area in the surgical arena, and double check with the person who comes to take the patient into the operating room to be sure he has the intended person for the specific doctor. If a surgeon has his own team he should have them, down to the orderlies, trained to think in terms of eliminating errors and making an open-minded game of being correct. If the surgeon works with one anesthesiologist most of the time, the anesthesiologist should be involved in the avoidance of surgical mistakes, like operating on the wrong patient, or the wrong side, or the wrong limb.

Too often in big open-staff hospitals, the surgeon takes the crew assigned to him at any particular time of the day in a busy schedule, and might walk into an operating room staffed with people unfamiliar with his routine. Some surgeons who have an itinerate practice, hopping from one hospital to another across the city, always in a hurry, might phone ahead and want the patient asleep and ready to go when he gets to the operating room. The operating room staff, hospital administration, the anesthesiologist, all should stand firm in not allowing this practice. It is fraught with the danger of error, like putting the wrong patient to sleep. And what if the surgeon has a wreck or a flat tire?

One remedy for these errors lies in the hands of the patient and his guardian, family or otherwise. What can anyone do to protect himself and to help improve the system? First, don't roll over and surrender personal rights, but be sensible. Adjust to the system as long as it does no harm. In the office and waiting room situation, take along paper work or a book and expect to wait. Write or telephone days ahead and ask for all forms to be mailed so they can be completed at home. The facts and concerns and questions about new symptoms or a new medical episode since the last appointment might be recorded and mailed ahead. If there for a routine evaluation only, and the doctor is behind schedule because he has had to attend to an emergency, or someone in the office has become an emergency, a waiting patient might volunteer to come back when the office is not harassed and overloaded. Signs of unprofessional conduct, like loitering, too much loud laughter, joke telling in the passageways, familiarities between nurses and the doctors, give any patient a good reason to leave and not come back.

Deeper into the system, the hospital patient or a responsible advocate, if possible both, need to be alert to the possibilities for error. Even with precautions, the matter of correct identity of person, drugs, procedures, and treatment haunts every patient in the medical system. Deadly mix-ups can and do occur in every department of a hospital, from bed to laboratory. The patients and the families can do much to help eliminate this fault by being vigilant in constant attendance at the bedside, by checking all labels, intended treatments, laboratory procedures, and reports.

CHILDREN

Children are people, too, real people, and to be called kid is to be diminished and insulted. To be treated in the spirit of the name is to be deprived of full recognition as a burgeoning human. Some adults choose to pass off the name as an expression of fondness, but to catch all its real meaning just listen to the use of the term. It means the opposite, more like my burden of secondary importance and my after thought. Why not call them what they are: children, my children, my family, my boys, my girls, or my boys and girls?

As we extend the formal education of our children, we delay their maturity. Proof of adult capabilities at an early age is apparent in street children of this world where in a struggle to live they practice all the adult enterprises from good to the worst, among them, hard work, stealing, robbery, murder, prostitution, and begging. They do it because this is their legacy from the world ruled by adults, their only way to survive. Left on their own, free of social and economic impediments of the modern educational system, children would grow to full-blown adult behavior at a much earlier age.

When children get sick, their illnesses are not of secondary importance. The child is something other than the simplistic concept of a small adult. The metabolism, physiology, digestion in particular, and the brain all have yet to mature to adult levels of function. Some of the roughage eaten by adults and often forced on the children is indigestible in their maturing gut. Most of their illnesses are minor, but parents should be alert for something worse. The fever and flu-like symptoms can turn to a violent and rapidly fatal illness in the course of a few hours, like the highly contagious and very lethal meningococcal meningitis, generally known as spinal meningitis. The pediatrician's job is not an enviable one. Any parent needs to call him again, despite his reassurances of "something going around," if the child's symptoms are growing worse.

In past generations childhood diseases and other health problems carried a high mortality, and survival of an entire family of children to adulthood was more the exception than otherwise. Infections took most of them. In the days before the germ theory and modern hygiene, old grandmothers and other women often chewed the food then fed it to infants who were having feeding problems. They did not recognize the possible harm from poor oral hygiene and diseases such as tuberculosis.

Drug dosage for children has to be adjusted not only to body size and age, but also to the effects on the growing body. Accidents and mistakes are more prone to occur if pediatrics is a division of a general hospital with common pharmacy and operating rooms for both children and adults. The child, too, needs family at the hospital bedside to guard against mistakes, as it should be guarded at home against drugs and household chemicals, loaded guns, dangerous knives, electric sockets, and other sources of injury.

Major birth defects should be operated on when they are a threat to survival and normal growth. Certain others, such as a sternum deformity, may not really need to be operated on if they will never compromise an otherwise normal life. A child in adolescence is old enough to help make the decision, and should be reassured about his appearance, even though it may deviate from the average.

Child abuse, whether mental, physical, verbal, or sexual, is one of humanity's greatest crimes. An infant expresses discomfort, distress, and hunger by crying. Speechless at birth and for months afterward, it has no other means of getting the necessary attention. The words, "spoiled rotten," are too often used as a shortcut to slapping, spanking, shaking, and other forms of violence. A careful look will always find reason for the squalling: an open safety pin, burning skin inside a soiled wet diaper, hunger, belly pain from gas, bug bites, too hot, too cold, clothes too tight, fever and other symptoms of illness, undetected injuries, and fright. "Spare the rod and spoil the child" is another excuse supported by religious authority. In response to such ignorance, it is safe to say the adult who strikes a child is a nasty-tempered coward out of control. A child once whipped by an angry parent will never be the same again and will carry hostility and resentment for the rest of his life.

For example, suppose you, a full grown adult, have a weak stomach for collard greens. A 15-foot giant, who has control over you, says, "Eat your collards." You won't eat your collards because you will get gas and a bellyache all night, and you don't like the taste. The giant smacks you a hard, openhanded blow across the face and forces you to eat the collards. Are you hurt? Are you angry? Damn right you are, and if you could fight back, you would. So how does the poor little child feel when he gets the same treatment? What does he carry in his heart, trapped in a world of adults? Violence under the guise of parental duty is simply a short cut to control. Reasoning and listening to the child's side of the situation take more time and patience. And on the part of the adult, it would take more respect for the significance of the child.

Guilty adults, parents, or foster parents will bring a battered child to the emergency room many months after the abuse has become serious. Their explanation of the injuries often is transparent, as in this case of a 3-and-a-half-year-old brought in because he had fallen from his high chair and bumped his head. The pitiful thing was unconscious, his head enlarged, the pupils of his eyes open and the optic nerve (nerves of sight) heads dead from chronic increased pressure inside the skull. Both arms and legs were fractured and deformed with big knobs of bone growth at the site of untreated breaks. There were healed craters of gouged-out flesh in his arms legs and belly and back, and open bleeding gouged-out craters scattered among the healed. He had fresh bleeding tooth sockets and healed tooth sockets, swollen puffy skin of the body and legs, bruises of every shade from red to black and green and yellow over the body and limbs, and swollen puffy blue-blotched scalp.

Emergency treatment included drainage of the clots from the compressed brain, but the child remained severely retarded and blind with chronic seizures due to brain damage, and spent the remainder of his shortened life in a state institution.

In no way could these injuries have been caused by a single fall from a high chair. The bone calluses at the fracture sites, the healed craters in flesh of the body and gums had to be near six months old. Destruction of sight from increased pressure in the head and the build up of chronic blood clots over the brain takes weeks or longer. Bruises turn different shades of color as days and weeks go by.

Police investigation found movies made by neighbors. These showed the child normal, active and pedaling a tricycle at Christmas time in the home of his foster parents. Then the real father of the child by a mistress took the boy home to his real wife. In seven months, the child had been ruined.

This case is just one among too many, a frequent emergency room customer. Child abuse is a far more common social ill than generally recognized. To not discover this cause of injury early on is to condemn the victim to increasing and protracted violence.

Chapter Six
VIGILANCE, DOUBLE-CHECKING RECORDS REPORTS

REPORTS AND CHARTS

Dr. Robert Gordon walked into one of his examining rooms and opened the chart in his hands. The patient had been waiting awhile. The doctor looked up and started talking. He did not know the patient's name until he read it off the record. Dr. Gordon did not have the gift of remembering names, or names and faces together, nor had he been trained to it. His questions didn't sound right to the patient, who hesitated in order to give Dr. Gordon a chance.

"How much insulin are you taking?"

"None," the patient answered.

Dr. Gordon wanted to know why not, indignation rising in his tone. How dare a patient disobey his doctor? Then he asked about blood sugar levels, and whether the patient was measuring twice a day. The patient had never measured his blood sugar and the last test, done the previous year during routine annual laboratory work, revealed entirely normal results. Something was wrong.

Had Dr. Gordon gone bonkers, or was the patient some kind of smartass giving him a bad time? The doctor folded the chart and read the cover, looked at the patient, looked at the chart again, and stormed out. A murmur of voices occurred in the hallway before the doctor returned with another chart in hand.

Dozens of people with the same or a similar name, like Tom Jones, Ben Williams, Susie Smith, etc., frequent any busy office. In this instance, the office help handed Dr. Gordon the wrong chart, and under pressure to get the work done, he did not double check before talking. He had only embarrassed himself in the situation, and chances were he would never be caught again in such a mistake. But under different circumstances such an error can be carried to grievous or fatal consequences. It happens all the time in hospitals and offices.

For example in this case Eric Simpson, a very dedicated and competent neurosurgeon, had just finished an eight-hour operation on a 50-year-old man, Tom Williams, to remove a large benign brain tumor, a meningioma. Dr. Simpson successfully got the entire tumor without damaging underlying and surrounding brain. Exhausted but elated, he went to the waiting room to inform the Williams family and to give them the good news. To his surprise, he found the patient's wife distraught and crying. Papa had incurable cancer of the lung. Someone had shown a member of the family the X-ray report on the record. Dr. Simpson's solar plexus took a nosedive. He had looked at the chest

X-ray pictures himself before surgery. How could he have missed it? He had seen no evidence of a growth. What was wrong here?

He excused himself and rushed back to the operating room, where the patient's X-ray film jacket with all the pictures waited for return to the radiology department. The nurses were still cleaning the room. He took the chest X-ray picture and popped it on the view box. There it was, a huge mass filling most of one lung, with a pool of fluid collected over the lower portion of the chest cavity. How could he have missed it? Simpson would never have put the patient through such a harrowing operation had he known of the fatal lung lesion. He stood there in near shock with shame and regret and confusion, looking at the picture.

But something seemed puzzling. This did not look like Tom William's chest. Then he saw the real picture. Tom Williams had grown two large breasts. Simpson found the patient's chart in the recovery room. The report of the chest X-ray picture on Mr. Williams described normal findings. Another chest X-ray report in the record described the malignant lung tumor, in the chest of a woman named Thelma Williams. Apparently, a mix-up had occurred in the radiology department. Had the radiologist goofed? Had the person who typed the report switched names accidentally? Dr. Simpson confronted the radiologist and left the problem there to be corrected. Some protective measures will be discussed in the chapter on X-ray departments.

Another depressing situation made the national news recently. Several days after a 48-year-old woman had both breasts removed, she was informed of a mistake in the diagnosis. She didn't have cancer of the breast after all. The tissue from the biopsy of her breast lesion had been switched with another person's. The other person had the cancer.

In the chain of events carrying this biopsy specimen from the operating room through the laboratory process, more than one person could be at fault. The surgeon himself should have gone to the laboratory and asked to see the slides of the biopsied material from the patient whose breasts he was about to remove. If he did examine the slides himself, did he check the numbers on the slides and match them with the correct name? The mistake was caught ultimately, but how? When something so drastic is to be done, the surgeon needs to look more carefully, or if in doubt go back to the previously biopsied lesion and get a frozen section and wait the few minutes for the results before proceeding. Caution and double-checking could have prevented the tragic mistake in this path of mammography and cautionary biopsy. The unfortunate woman paid a terrible price for trusting the system.

So, how can people stop such terrible mistakes from happening to themselves or members of their families? At first it may seem like an impossible task, but only if the patient and all concerned surrender to the system. No one should accept bad news until he sees the evidence.

Ask to be shown the slides, have the malignancy pointed out, double check the identifying numbers on the slides and on the patient's chart. Before giving up both breasts, ask for a second biopsy, a second opinion, or both, and don't be panicked into rash decisions. Think in terms of raw reality. Chances are this woman would not have let this man even touch her breasts had he not been her doctor, yet she let him cut both off without putting up any kind of fight. Patients, for their own good, have to learn to question the system.

All unfavorable findings should be double, even triple checked by the doctor before reporting to a patient or a family, and the family and patient should be skeptical about accepting an unfavorable report until they are convinced it is true. Every precaution against mistakes should be made before submitting to disfiguring and deforming surgery.

VIGILANCE: WATCH THE PATIENT

An alert doctor can avert a tragedy, as happened in the following case at a southern university hospital during the days before CAT scanners and the MRI. During a quiet lull near twilight, an ambulance brought a young man, a carpenter, to the emergency room. No family came with him. According to the ambulance attendants the patient fell off a roof and was unconscious at first, but had awakened en route. The emergency room personnel called the neurosurgery service. Evaluation showed a knot beneath a scalp bruise in the right temple. The patient was groggy but seemed to be improving. X-ray pictures of the skull revealed a hairline crack through the right temporal bone, in front of the ear, beneath the region of the bruise. The pictures also showed a round white speck about a quarter inch in diameter right in the middle of the skull cavity just behind the ear region. This was a normal finding, due to calcium deposits in the pineal gland, and it reliably identifies the middle of the skull cavity. The pineal gland is part of the brain, and if anything pushes the brain to one side, the pineal image shifts with it. The attending doctors had gone home for the evening, leaving the neurosurgical resident in charge. He decided to watch the patient carefully because the skull crack crossed the course of a small artery passing from beneath the scalp through the skull to supply the major brain cover, the dura. Such injuries often tear the artery, leading to hemorrhage between bone and the dura, forming a rapidly expanding clot compressing the brain and quickly progressing to coma and death if not promptly and correctly treated.

The patient was confused enough to be difficult and insisted on going home. The doctor, concerned about possible complications, refused and told him he would be kept in the emergency room for observation. The resident then left to make evening hospital rounds with his entourage of assistants and medical students. A few minutes into his rounds, he was paged by the ER nurse. The patient's family was signing him out of the hospital. "Who is?" asked the resident. His brother and sister, the nurse informs him. The doctor asked their ages. "Fifteen and 16," she replied.

"They can't sign him out. They are minors."

"They insist," she said.

"No way," he said. "Send them home to get their parents."

"They live out in the country."

"Good," he said. "We will have control over the situation longer, maybe long enough to see what's going to happen."

While the conversation continued, the patient was getting rowdier and cursing, and insisting on going home. "I'll be back down in a few minutes," the resident told the nurse. The resident was paged again in another 15 minutes. The patient was getting drowsy. The resident instructed the nurse to order another X-ray picture of the skull and called the operating room to get ready. The resident's entourage arrived as the new X-ray picture came out of the developing vat. The calcified pineal had shifted two centimeters to the left. The patient had become very drowsy, silent, and offered no resistance to treatment. They rushed him to surgery, drilled a hole through the skull in front of the ear, and evacuated the clot. The patient was alert and cooperative a few minutes later when the orderlies removed him from the operating table to a stretcher.

This patient would have died had he been allowed to check himself out of the hospital in his state of growing confusion. Here an alert doctor perhaps encroached on a patient's rights, but he recognized faulty judgment aggravated by the head injury.

Here is another real one. A tube passed down the windpipe between the vocal cords makes anesthesia safer when used correctly, especially when breathing has been paralyzed deliberately with drugs. Then breathing has to be done with a machine or by hand-squeezing a bag attached to the tube. This requires an airtight fit of the tube in the throat. Most tubes have a balloon near the tip, and this balloon is inflated after the tube has been placed. Accidents happen with this arrangement. People forget to deflate the balloon before removal of the tube, and damage the vocal cords.

Anesthesia hit on a safer idea. Use the tube without a balloon and pack around it with wet gauze for an airtight fit above the vocal cords. In this particular incidence, a patient was brought to the recovery room with the balloon-less tube still in place, waiting for the anesthesia to lighten. They took the patient off the gurney, pulled him over in bed, and a nurse removed the tube. Immediately the patient started a muffled coughing spasm, began to gag, and turned blue in the face. An intern had the presence of mind to look in the throat, saw a tag of gauze, reached in with a clamp and pulled out the material. He retrieved about 15 feet of narrow, wet, gauze binding. The patient began to breathe normally. Had the intern not been present and savvy, the patient would have choked to death quickly.

The remedy here is more elusive: In neither of these cases could a member of the family have been present. In the first, the family had to be found and notified. The employer should have had someone there to look after the man injured on the job, and he surely would have insisted on the patient's remaining in the hospital in the presence of his irrational behavior. In the second, no family member is likely to be allowed in the recovery room of a busy operating suite. In certain situations, like the second incident, a family can't do much. However, if a person is turning blue in the face and gagging after the removal of an endotracheal tube, anyone should know to look down the throat for the culprit. These two cases simply help paint the picture of the real world of medicine.

Chapter Seven
DRUGS, ANESTHESIA, AND GASES

DRUGS

The ***Journal of the American Medical Association*** reported a study of 1994 statistics pointing to adverse prescription drug reaction as the fourth- to sixth-leading cause of death in the United States, a total of 106,000 people. A University of Toronto study of 33 million patients admitted to American hospitals in 1994 reported more than 100,000 deaths from drugs administered either before or after hospitalization, with another two million patients suffering side effects. Current reports do nothing to change this grim picture.

These studies examine causes, among them adverse reactions between mixtures. For example, antihistamines in combination with some antibiotics lead to abnormal and sometimes fatal heart reaction. Certain drugs carry a lethal potential secondary to the intended effect. For instance, blood thinners might cause spontaneous and fatal internal hemorrhage. The studies also point to the lack of sufficient knowledge about all the actions of any given drug alone, and in combination with other drugs.

Drug mishaps account for the greatest number of accidental deaths in the medical system. The wrong drug, wrong dose, wrong patient, wrong route of administration, adverse reaction with another drug, and allergic reactions lie at the root of most of the errors.

Here is an example of a drug mishap. Back in 1943, the dean of a small southern medical school, lecturing to the second-year students on some of the practices and safeguards in medicine, told of deforming one of his patients by an accident with drugs. He was a very competent eye, ear, nose, and throat doctor, who passed on a great legacy in medicine to his children and grandchildren, who themselves now are famous in medicine. He told the class, "Don't ever administer a drug in any form unless you yourself have taken it out of the manufacturer's container after reading and double checking all labels." Then he told the class what had happened to him as a young doctor when he let his guard down for a minute.

He asked his nurse for Argyrol, a relatively mild silver colloidal suspension used to treat conjunctivitis in the days before antibiotics. She passed him pure silver nitrate instead, and he had already dropped a drop onto the waiting and trusting eye before the patient's violent reaction showed the nurse's error. Despite instant emergency measures, the cornea was scarred and the white of the eye (sclera) turned permanently a shade of gray. The moral he presented was simply never to accept and use an unlabeled drug or chemical from other hands.

The frankness of this highly respected physician and teacher served as a guide to ethical and professional behavior of these young men, his students, throughout their careers.

Another example occurred more than 50 years ago in a famous university hospital where ruptured lumbar (low back) discs were customarily operated on under spinal anesthesia with the patient in the face down position. Before starting the operation, the surgeon would routinely supplement the spinal anesthesia by injecting Novocain in the midline skin of the low back at the site of the incision, a place where the spinal anesthetic left some sensitivity. The surgeon accepted a syringe of Novocain from his scrub nurse. She was the best, but she had a waspish disposition. As she handed him the syringe of clear fluid with needle mounted, he asked, "Is this Novocain?"

"What the hell you think it is … alcohol?"

He injected the fluid into the skin, puffing it up, and the tissue turned a peculiar chalk-white almost instantly, and then began to darken. The surgeon stopped and sniffed the syringe. It was indeed alcohol. Alcohol kills and preserves tissue. He at once picked up a scalpel and made an elliptical excision of the injected area, removing a piece of skin and the underlying tissue as big as a medium sized banana. He wrapped the material in a gauze pad and discarded it in the waste bucket. After the operation had been completed, the ruptured disc material successfully removed, the surgeon closed the skin easily by undermining both sides of the incision, creating slack to make up for the lost tissue.

Nothing was ever said about this incident outside the operating room. The patient got well and never knew the difference. This accident happened because the operating room personnel broke the cautionary rules. The scrub nurse in question kept two small stainless steel cups on her table. In preparing for surgery, the circulating nurse would fill one with Novocain from the supply bottle and the other with alcohol. During surgery, the scrub nurse wet sponges in the alcohol and used them to wipe blood off the instruments passed from the operation onto the instrument tray. The two solutions were both clear fluids.

In preparing for the operation, the scrub nurse had aspirated alcohol instead of Novocain into the syringe, and her irritated response to the surgeon's cautious question kept her from thinking. Medicine is no place to wear your pride. The scrub nurse herself should always have aspirated the Novocain, or any other material for injection into a patient, from the manufacturer's bottle herself. Better, the surgeon himself should aspirate the fluid to be injected into his patient. This is a striking example of system failure.

Here is another. The brain and the spinal cord and its connections float in and contain a clear liquid called spinal fluid. About 150cc (roughly half a cup) is produced by the nervous system per day. Normally, this enclosed circulating fluid system is water tight and airtight. Occasionally, it springs a leak, usually where the front lobes of the brain rest just above a portion of the skull floor full of holes (the cribriform plate), through which many branches of the olfactory (smell) nerve go into the lining of the nose. Spontaneously or following a blow to the head, an unusual amount of fluid begins to ooze, maybe even drip, from the nose. Headaches may develop. The patient at first gets a lot of speculation and treatment for one thing or another, like bad cold, influenza, or allergic rhinitis. Someone finally thinks of spinal fluid. This is a dangerous situation, sometimes leading to fatal meningitis because germs can go right from the nose into the brain coverings. The doctor needs to know.

A continuous spinal fluid leak requires a major operation to reestablish barriers against the outside world, but the diagnosis has to be correct and the approximate location of the opening identified. The neurosurgeon can employ one of several techniques to identify the nasal drainage as spinal fluid. The normal nasal discharge and spinal fluid have different chemical characteristics identifiable in the laboratory. Spinal fluid has a sugar level equal to the level carried by the bloodstream, and nasal discharge does not. If a dye is placed to color the circulating pool of spinal fluid, then the drainage coming out of the nose has the same color if it actually is spinal fluid. The doctor does this by performing a spinal tap and placing a harmless dye in the fluid at the level of the tap. Within a short time, colored fluid should come from the nose.

Performance of the test is usually relegated to one of the residents in training, like a junior assistant. It's supposed to be a very simple procedure. The harmless vegetable dye injected into the spinal fluid pathways is indigo carmine, and has an intense deep blue-green color. It has been used many times with no ill effects.

The doctor had the patient lying on his side on the table. The needle had been inserted at the midline of the low back into the spinal fluid pool. The nurse handed the doctor the syringe full of the green-blue fluid. He took it, removed the stylet from the spinal needle, watched the fluid drop from the needle, then injected the dye in one big dollop. Instantly the patient screamed and soon complained of his legs feeling dead. The process continued until within only a few minutes of the injection, the patient could not move his legs and could feel nothing in them, not even touch. The paralysis crept up to mid-chest level and became complete. In subsequent months and years the patient never improved.

The source of the dye was traced back to the supply from which it came. Instead of indigo carmine, the nurse had handed the doctor a syringe filled with methylene blue, an aniline dye of the about same color and extremely destructive to the nervous system. An investigation placed the blame on one of several people involved in the route of the methylene blue from its source in the supplies to the patient. Regardless of where the blame fell, this was another instance of failure of the system. It happened because the doctor did not aspirate the dye himself from a labeled bottle of indigo carmine. The doctor should have known better, but he would have had to have changed the way the system handled such procedures. He was young and inexperienced, not mature or not cynical enough yet to buck the system. And he broke yet another rule—when injecting anything other than an inoculation, a small amount should be tried first. If no reaction occurs, then proceed.

The dismal parade of cases goes on, some with modern drugs, some with drugs in use for decades. As reported in the national news, a 7-year-old Florida boy died from an attempted elective ear operation. The surgeon injected a local anesthetic containing a blood vessel constrictor (epinephrine, also called adrenaline) into the skin at the operative site to supplement the general anesthesia and to help control bleeding. The patient quickly developed heart problems and died the next day. Extensive investigation revealed Epinephrine (adrenaline) 1/1000 instead of a mixture of Lidocaine one percent with Epinephrine 1/100,000 had been handed to the surgeon. The circulating nurse and an assistant had been given the responsibility for mixing the drug combination before surgery. It was the hospital's way of doing things, and the death changed the routine without question. Such mixtures should come from pharmacy and not be trusted to anyone outside pharmacy, or better yet, they should come directly from the manufacturer. The surgeon himself should aspirate the drug from the original container as he reads the label.

Although a patient could have done little to stop any of these accidents, these cases do set out the cardinal rule for doctor and patient alike: Never use a drug from an unlabeled container. The same applies to the medications at home. Never mix them in a common container, and never take a pill from an unlabeled bottle.

In certain situations, someone should intercede on the side of caution. A nurse enters the hospital room with a tray on which rest three syringes of clear fluid, unlabeled, with needles mounted, two of them for patients farther down the hall. Beware! Refuse to submit to the injection. One of these could very well be a poison if given to the wrong patient, probably none of them harmful if the right medicine goes to the right person, but her technique invites mistakes, and mistakes with drugs too often are fatal. This cannot be said too many times or emphasized too strongly—*the person administering the drug should always take it directly from the labeled container in the presence of the patient.* Storage in the same shelf area of two or more frequently used and potentially dangerous drugs can lead to misuse of one or all.

Accidents happen at the site of injections. The chosen sites include in the skin and under the skin (subcutaneous), into the muscle, or into a blood vessel. Drugs designated for the first or second site should not be injected into the bloodstream. Small doses of rapidly absorbed drugs go under the skin, larger deposits to be absorbed over a period of time are placed deep into a muscle layer. These are big doses and may have an oil base. They certainly should not go directly into the blood, where they could prove to be fatal.

Technique for deep injections is all-important. The needle should be inserted quickly and kindly. The plunger should be pulled back to be sure the needle tip is not in a blood vessel. The injection should be slow. Rapid injections split the tissue and can be quite painful. The injection should not damage hidden structures. Serious damage to the sciatic and the radial nerves is common. The radial nerve courses around the back of the upper arm below shoulder level and down toward the front of the elbow. If the nurse approaches the back of the arm just below the shoulder, stop her. The injection should be in the deltoid muscle, on the outer area just below the shoulder joint. A radial nerve injection will cause a wrist drop, a very disabling injury, and it may not be repairable.

The sciatic nerve courses through the middle of the cheek of the buttock and down the back of the thigh. When a person sits down, he sits right over the course of this nerve. Injections should be done in the upper outer quadrant of a buttock. Two or three ccs of an oil-based drug injected directly into a sciatic nerve wreaks havoc. The foot is paralyzed for motion up and down; some of the leg muscles are paralyzed; sensory loss is profound, and pain sometimes unbearable. The damage is too extensive for repair and at best the results are never good enough. Call the nurse on it, slow her down, make her think and double check, and ignore the huffy response. Her position is not defensible.

The wrong drug dosage can be fatal or cause major problems. Blood thinners, like heparin and Coumadin (warfarin) are notorious causes of drug accidents. The wrong dose can lead to damaging or fatal hemorrhage and the type of stroke due to bleeding into the brain.

Here is an example of complications with a blood thinner. On the grounds of a southern university hospital, a carpenter accidentally cut off one of his thumbs with a power saw. A savvy fellow, he picked up the thumb and ran for the emergency room. The hand surgeon came down from his clinic immediately, took the patient to the operating room, and reattached the thumb, an operation requiring several hours because of the necessity to sew tiny arteries and veins and nerves, a very tedious procedure done under magnification. These arteries and veins are not easy to keep open. They clot off almost certainly unless an anticoagulant (blood thinner) is administered constantly in drip form until the danger has passed. The surgeon wrote an order for a heparin drip, with the dosage and drip rate spelled out. The surgeon returned to the clinic to see the waiting patients he had to leave for the emergency, and a couple of hours went by. Then he had a call from the floor nurse. His patent was bleeding too much. The blood had dripped through the dressing which they had reinforced twice already to no avail. The surgeon walked on the ward, looked at the heparin drip, and immediately recognized the problem. A tenfold error had been made in pharmacy, and the error was evident in the label. He shut off the drip and ordered protamine to reverse the thinner, then asked the nurse to get the pharmacist down to the floor at once, and set about changing the dressing.

While the unsuspecting surgeon was busy, the pharmacist arrived and went to the pole holding the heparin container. He took the container down, unplugged the tubing at its point of entry into the container, and disappeared with labeled bag. No one has been able to find the stolen container to this day, and the pharmacist denies the error. The patient went back to surgery, the wound opened to remove accumulated blood clot, the operation done over, but ischemic (without blood) time had been too long. Within days the thumb turned black and had to be removed. The surgeon months later transplanted one of the patient's big toes to the thumb base to give the patient some semblance of prehensile skill in the hand, a long and painful and expensive operation, with the added cost of a lame foot.

These multiple errors—the wrong drug dosage, then the sneaky act of hiding it—point to faults in the system. Until finger pointing and blame placing are taken from the system, it will continue to malfunction under such circumstances. At the bedside immediately after surgery, a family member who questioned everything might have caught the dosage error by reading the label, but such ability to intervene is asking too much of the average family.

A mandatory and ritualistic double-checking of the figures on the drug label and the figures written by the surgeon would have prevented the accident. Personnel working in the system brought the container to the ward, hung it on the pole, and turned the controls on. No one double-checked the label. And a savvy family member would have stopped the thief.

The preceding cases all have dealt with mix-ups in drug identity and dosage. These are preventable human errors. Deeper into drug problems, the hazards are not so easily identified or so simple to remedy. Here in the early years of the twenty-first century, the ignorance of the ultimate effects of adding more chemicals (drugs) to the complex biochemistry of the human body far exceeds the vital wisdom and understanding necessary to safety. Witness the harm and the litigation now erupting from the use of drugs highly touted by the drug industry. No doubt this situation will improve with time and experience. But almost any substance known to man is poisonous if taken in excessive amounts or by the wrong route, and this is true even of water. A person who drinks too much of it without getting an adequate supply of electrolytes like sodium and potassium, and foods like glucose, gets sick. Yet, a person can drink many glasses of pure water without doing real harm, while only a small amount injected into a vein can be fatal. For this reason, solutions fed through the veins must have carefully balanced contents. An element critical to life at a certain level can become lethal at a higher level. Potassium is a striking example. Too low a level weakens heart muscle, leading to heart failure. Too much stops the heart.

Potassium chloride (KCL) is a component of most life-sustaining intravenous solutions used in the hospitals. It must be mixed into the entire volume of the container of solution, and thus diluted to a safe level. This mixing, safer done in the pharmacy, would be safest in prepackaged intravenous preparations from the manufacturer. But this is what can happen. A doctor walks into an intensive care unit (ICU), reads the lab reports on his patient's chart and finds the potassium level too low. He writes an order for a vial of potassium chloride. The nurse obeys the order incorrectly, injecting the potassium directly into the tube toward the vein, and the patient dies. Had the same amount been placed in and mixed with the bag of solution, the potassium would have been properly diluted. Potassium chloride, besides its great value to life, is also one of the three drugs in the executioner's mixture, responsible for stopping the heart.

Because of its vital role in sustaining life, potassium chloride is commonplace in hospital pharmacies and on the supply shelves of the wards, and due to its ready accessibility, has become the source of fatal hospital mistakes. It should be injected directly into the blood only for the purpose of execution.

When a person comes in the patient's room and begins getting ready to inject something into the IV tubing or directly into a vein, the patient or his guardian should find out what the nurse intends to inject before she proceeds. Let her know someone knows how potassium chloride is correctly administered. Furthermore, she just might be in the wrong room. It happens!

Cumulative effects of drugs may be deceptive and often fatal. Tragedy can strike someone who is walking about at work as it did to this unfortunate young man, the senior resident in urology at a university hospital. It happened on Thanksgiving morning many years ago, while he was making hospital rounds with several nurses, medical students, and younger residents. At the foot of a patient's bed he gurgled in the middle of a sentence, turned blue in the face, and suddenly collapsed. Two resident doctors broke his fall, and resuscitation attempts were immediate and vigorous, but he was already dead. Everyone was astounded and puzzled. The promising young man had nearly finished his training and was scheduled to join his older brother already well established in a huge urology practice in New Orleans. He had a beautiful young wife, two children, a boy and girl, and a very favorable future. There had to be an explanation.

The autopsy revealed no cause for sudden death, the heart normal, Contrary to expectations. His family had to accept the puzzling conclusion of **natural death**. Complete studies in the hospital laboratory on his blood samples found no toxins, but samples were sent to the state toxicologist for additional studies. The coroner, after two years studying the evidence and investigating the circumstances, made a diagnosis of death due to a combination of drugs. The young man was not an addict, but he was a closet alcoholic and had been fighting his problem with the help of medical treatment. The medical treatment along with the alcohol had led to cardiac arrest.

Sudden deaths in alcoholics are common. In the past, chloral hydrate and paraldehyde were used to control the manifestations of delirium tremens (the DTs). The combination of drugs and alcohol sometimes led to sudden death, especially when the doctor became discouraged with the effects of the sedatives and allowed the patient to have alcohol in an attempt to slow the DTs. The drugs used now (more than 20 benzodiazepines, like Valium) in the treatment of alcoholics carry some risk of sudden death.

A bad situation repeats itself in every hospital and town and community when several doctors are treating a patient at the same time, and not one takes the time to know what the others are doing. The patient might receive five or six or more different drugs from several doctors, and the results can be fatal or render life nearly intolerable, as it did to this 97-year-old woman who developed severe GI bleeding from the non-steroid anti-inflammatory drug, Nalfon, used at the time to treat macular degeneration. Instead of stopping the offending drug and treating the anemia, the doctor put her through a complete gastrointestinal (GI) workup—barium enema, barium swallow, gastroscopy, colonoscopy—and consultation with a general surgeon, consultation with a gastroenterologist, and she was seen by two of his associates. This evaluation continued for a week during which time the anemia was not treated, the patient became more exhausted, and complained of pain in her arthritic spine. Five different doctors wrote orders for five different drugs (Haldol, Demerol, Mellaril, Ambien, and Ativan). None of them paid any attention to the drugs already ordered by the other doctors. The patient became psychotic, hallucinated, climbed over the top of the side rails and fell to the floor, sustaining a broken sternum, fractured ribs, a broken hip, loss of bowel and bladder control, and became dangerously ill with pneumonia and a raging bladder infection. She had walked into the hospital on her cane, and she never walked again and never went home. She died in a nursing home seven years later.

This is not the only case of its kind, nor is it the entire story. It shows this terrible dilemma of modern life. The arrogance of the system is maddening, and the victims helpless, unless a caring family intervenes to stop such mistreatments. Similar circumstances develop in nursing homes by the hundreds throughout this wealthy land. Our society allows the care of the disabled and the elderly to be a profit-making business, existing solely to make money for the investors. The primary function is not the care of the patients. In the interest of profit, not enough adequately trained people are hired to take care of the patient load. It would cost too much and cut too deeply into profits. The nursing shortage in general is due to job elimination by these very restrictions.

As a result, a person in a nursing home or the hospital needs daily attention from the family or from someone there for the family. Otherwise, the truly disabled will die sooner. In hospitals and nursing homes, drugs too often are used to shut the patient up, not to treat the illness causing the misery, discomfort, and noisy behavior.

The remedy calls for alertness, knowledge, and meticulous care. The numerous causes of drug errors are related to the very complexity of the pharmacy system. Every drug has at least four names and sometimes more. A combination of drugs, concocted by different drug companies, will have another name calculated to stimulate sales. Many drugs have deceptively similar names and packaging.

Mixtures produce toxic reactions in one of several ways. **Additive** means effects equal to the sum of the effects of two or more chemicals. **Synergistic** means an effect greater than the sum of the drugs. **Potentiation** means increased toxic effect of one drug in the presence of a nontoxic one.

The patient needs to know whether such interaction occurs between any two drugs he might be taking. Paperback guides to prescription and non-prescription drugs are available at many bookstores. The **Physician's Desk Reference** (PDR) comes as near to being complete as any publication, but it is expensive. Fortunately, it is available in the reference section of most public libraries. It lists the complications of each drug, the drugs with which it reacts unfavorably, and the circumstances under which a person should not take it. This reference source is available also at **www.pdr.net**. Furthermore, information on any drug can be found by using an Internet search engine.

Certain foods increase the potency of some drugs, and others interfere with the desired drug action. The National Consumers League Web site (**www.nclnet.org**) has a wealth of information on this subject as well as information on the faults and dangers of some over-the-counter medications.

The doctor's handwriting often is a problem, and every nurse and pharmacist who has to tolerate this slovenliness should call the offender on his bad habits and get a correct interpretation. Abbreviations can lead to confusion of identity. Illegible prescriptions should be clarified before the patient leaves the doctor's office.

What can a patient or the patient's guardian do about drugs, in the hospital or out? Check the name, purpose, and the dosage. In the hospital, insist on having a list of the scheduled medications, and question anyone who enters the room with a variation of this regimen. Insist on knowing what is going on if anyone tries to inject something into the tube of an IV already in use.

In general, be wary of television ads. A given drug with a proprietary or brand name (copyrighted, patented, or trademarked) might cost much more than its generic counterpart. Tylenol is an example. Acetaminophen is its generic form and costs usually less than half as much. Tylenol is also a component in more than three hundred different compounds, each with its own mysterious name. A search of the latest editions of the foremost textbooks of pharmacology used in modern medical schools will reveal none of these Tylenol concoctions. Most of these mixtures are heavily advertised and recklessly touted. Acetaminophen relieves pain and lowers fever as will aspirin, but without many of the side effects. It is not a blood thinner, and it does not significantly decrease inflammation. It can damage the liver when used incorrectly.

The NSAIDs are the non-steroid anti-inflammatory drugs, aspirin being the oldest, the simplest, the least expensive, and often the least potentially harmful. The newer NSAIDs, some of which can be bought over the counter, are being blamed for an increasing number of deaths. Bleeding in the intestinal tract and fluid retention with rapid weight gain are two major complications. Heart damage from some of them is now a recognized hazard. Unfortunately, several of these drugs have come to be used carelessly to relieve simple pain when a less dangerous drug would suffice. Unless fighting inflammation, as in painful arthritis, a person does not need one of the powerful NSAIDs. When needed, this treatment should be under the supervision of a doctor. Its side effects can be fatal. The constant barrage of television hype about one or the other of these drugs and combinations thereof is unreliable. The claim of one type of pure acetaminophen or one type of pure aspirin being superior to another is false.

The recommendation of aspirin as a preventative measure against heart attack and stroke should be handled with reason. Stroke or heart attack in this instance means the blockage of a blood vessel due to a combination of disease in the arterial wall plus sludging or clotting in the blood flowing through the bad region. Aspirin inhibits the clotting mechanism in the bloodstream in a two-fold way. First, it destroys the chemical action responsible for platelets sticking together, and it destroys the second action of the same chemical, blood vessel constriction. Destruction of the first action is permanent for the remainder of the life of a platelet, a span of seven to 10 days. When taken as a preventative measure, small doses of aspirin are thought to be sufficient, 81mg per day (one pediatric-sized tablets) to 320 mg (5 grains, one adult tablet). Some physicians think one 81mg tablet a week is enough since the platelet lives only about seven days. Preventative doses are one thing; therapeutic doses are quite another and should be used under medical supervision. Excessive aspirin use leads to easy bleeding, bruises, and hemorrhages in the skin, and more serious complications like a bleeding type of stroke.

The world of drugs bewilders everyone, including doctors. Too often, a doctor's latest information has come from a detail man who presents information dictated by his employer, the drug company. A detail man sells the products of a drug manufacturer for whom he works. He supplies the physician's shelves with free samples. If such a drug gets passed on to a patient, a printed enclosure from the drug company should go along with it. Altogether, there are more than 10,000 drugs and drug concoctions on the market. This requires the careful use of reference books by both pharmacist and physician, and reading about each drug would be especially beneficial to the person taking the medicine. Many references are available, among them, **The Johns Hopkins Consumer Guide to Drugs.** Pull up any drug name on Google or another search engine, and a wealth of information is there instantly, like magic, in plain, understandable language.

Everything has its price. All medications for any one patient should be under the super vision and the coordination of one physician. The patient who buys an over-the-counter product without knowing all of its possible effects on the human body and takes it along with prescription drugs is playing a form of Russian roulette. If a person must attempt his own treatment, then he should do extensive reading in the available references, and shouldn't rely on word of mouth about chemicals available without a prescription.

Two recently published books, **The Truth About the Drug Companies** by Marcia Angell, M.D., and **Powerful Medicines** by Jerry Avorn, M.D. (see Bibliography), reveal the alarming tactics being used to victimize the public, you and me, and especially those who are less fortunate. These tactics have to do with money and politics. The full extent of this ugly situation is described in the books. The following are some of the findings summarized:

1. The FDA is not an all-powerful protective agency, and the public cannot always rely on it for safety. Approval of a drug may occur when a short clinical trial shows it to be superior to a placebo, or better than nothing. The trial may have lasted no more than a few weeks, and the drug does not have to be tested against the effectiveness of other drugs already on the market. On the Contrary, a drug may have been approved after a long period of evaluation, only to begin showing adverse effects after long usage.

2. The drug companies are now financing research in our academic institutions and exert monetary pressure to get the answers they want. Also, a pervasive influence is brought to bear on continued medical education, where drug companies fund, to different degrees, parties, banquets, and individual dinners. Hired agencies paid by a drug company plan medical meetings including the subject matter, speakers, and the results of research. Money calls the shots.

3. The wholesale cost of a drug is an arbitrary figure. The excuse of the high cost of research and development of new lifesaving drugs is not tenable when the cost of sales and advertising is a far larger figure for a particular drug. Money pours not into research so much as to promoting a drug of dubious superiority to one already on the market.

Near the time of a particular patent expiration, a drug company will alter the original molecular structure with a chemical short cut, give the results a new name, get a new patent, and sell the product at a high price. Prilosec and Nexium (the purple pill) are thus related. Prilosec retailed at six dollars a dose before the patent expired, and now can be bought for less than a dollar. Nexium costs four dollars and more, with no proven clinical superiority over Prilosec. The Claritin and Clarinex story is similar. The Claritin patent has expired, and the drug can be bought cheaply over the counter, in comparison to its former price and the cost of its newly patented successor, Clarinex. The liver converts Claritin to Clarinex, so taking the older drug produces the same effective agent. In moving another way around an expiring patent, a major drug company will pay another company not to produce and sell the medicine in its generic form. The authors of both cited books record these circumstances in detail.

4. Drug companies protect and advance themselves by a powerful Washington lobby. A congressman might come to represent the drug company interests, not his constituents, the patients. Congress has loosened the bonds on television advertising, and we hear only a few complications rattled off almost too fast to comprehend while the television shill touts us to "Ask your doctor about so and so." This technique is used to push drugs offering no special advantage over less expensive and sometimes better preparations of a drug, perhaps after decades of use, or even centuries of use, as with the aspirin.

A variety of drugs or drug mixtures of various mysterious names, each pushed by a different company, may all have essentially the same action.

5. The number of suitable patients for a particular clinical trial may be scarce, so the drug companies recruit volunteers through a variety of tactics including payments from a few hundred to a few thousand dollars each. Doctors are also paid by the drug companies and by contract research organizations hired by the companies for recruiting. These companies pay as much as several thousand dollars for each patient, then a large bonus for an extra, like the sixth person. The doctor prescribes for a patient the red or green pill at several dollars each. This automatically enrolls the patient in the so-called clinical evaluation, and the patient might not be aware of the action. The doctor gets paid sometimes as much as $7,000 to $12,000 for using the patient's name, sometimes as much as $30,000 for an extra bonus patient. The patient pays the high price, though the generic predecessor of the new pill is just as effective and costs far less. The patient is not getting the new medicine because it is better, but because it is a part of a multimillion-dollar marketing push, and the doctor and his office staff have been visited, entertained, indoctrinated, and snow-jobbed by the detail man. This system induces the enrollment of patients not suited to the study. For instance, a patient might be labeled asthmatic for a study while presenting no evidence of asthmatic disease.

On the academic scene, the need for enrollment in clinical trials exerts significant financial pressure on academic evaluation of results and the choice of treatment. Medical schools desperate for funding are falling into the clutches of commerce. The sponsors expect decisions favorable to their commercial interests.

6. Citizens of the United States pay higher prices for drugs than do patients in any other country. The discrepancy does not end there. Large groups like the Veterans Administration and HMOs can buy the drugs at a lower cost, but individuals cannot. The burden for full price falls on those least able to pay: the old, uninsured, and financially deprived. A bill introduced in 2003 establishing drug coverage under Medicare forbids government negations for lower drug costs. At present the system is in a state of disarray, with numerous confusing insurance plans competing for the patient dollar and a confounding failure in drug delivery. To summarize briefly, the drug industry is creeping toward a position of control by financing the institutions responsible for monitoring their behavior through scientific investigation of the products.

The Angell and Avorn books are recommended reading for anyone who wants to work toward improving the system.

So, what can we do about the prescription drug problem? The citizens of this country have become angry enough twice in the last hundred years to bring about radical changes to right the wrongs being done by the reckless tactics of big business. In 1906, Upton Sinclair's novel **The Jungle** aroused President Theodore Roosevelt and the people behind him to stop unrestrained practices in the meat packing industry. This gave rise to the Food and Drug Administration and the first controls on food and drugs sold to the public. In the early twenty-first century, telemarketers irritated too many people, and pressure on congress defeated the lobbyists and severely hampered the annoying practice. Now a third attack is overdue, this time on out-of-control behavior in the name of greed. It is time for every congressman to hear from his constituents loud and clear about the pervasive influence of health insurance and drug industry lobbies. Drugs for the elderly, nursing home care for the destitute, and medical treatment for the indigent should be motivated by more than profit for the investors. We as a nation should be ashamed to allow profit to take precedence over care of our old people who are unable to live at home with their families. Cost-cutting tactics on the care of senior citizens are comparable to the pre-FDA days in the food and drug industries. Congress needs to do something about drug problems and the out-of-hand insurance industry (see Chapter 16).

ANESTHESIA

Local anesthesia usually is administered by the surgeon with the exception of local blocks of large areas such as one limb or another in preparation for surgery with the patient awake. General anesthesia falls into other hands. Lucky indeed is the patient who has a competent, dedicated anesthesiologist throughout an operation. This person holds life and future well-being in his hands from beginning to the end of the procedure. All his moments are precarious. The surgeon, on the Contrary, most likely will have only a few moments of critical activity where failure could cost a life.

An anesthesiologist is a medical doctor trained in anesthesiology. An anesthetist is someone else, usually a registered nurse, trained in anesthesia. Nurse anesthetists bore the brunt of anesthesia responsibilities in this country through most of the twentieth century as the specialty of anesthesiology grew. Today, first-rate hospitals have a full staff of anesthesiologists. Others have a skeletal staff assigned to supervise a team of nurse anesthetists. The degree of excellence and safety depends on the commitment of the doctors in anesthesia. Nurse anesthetists usually are excellent, but they do not carry the authority of an anesthesiologist if something goes wrong. Aside from the surgery itself, the patient's best chances of coming out of an operation unscathed lie with the anesthesiologist who begins with the patient and stays with the patient until he is awake and safe again. An anesthesiologist supervising a team of anesthetists in one room might be too occupied with a critical problem to respond quickly enough to a second emergency elsewhere.

Every anesthetic agent in common use is a deadly poison, but a combination of these drugs used at sublethal levels usually produces a satisfactory anesthetic state with reasonable safety, as long as a knowledgeable person constantly monitors the patient. A good anesthesiologist knows physiology, metabolism, and drugs—especially drugs—and medicine in general as does no one else. He takes a person down through the shades of sleep toward death to spare unbearable pain. Oxygen level, carbon dioxide level, blood pressure, sugar level, temperature level, blood volume, urinary drainage, anesthetic level, electrolyte level, breathing, and heart rate must all be controlled. This requires constant attention to monitoring devices and to the patient's condition.

If the anesthesiologist is given to careless habits like going out in the hallway to talk on a phone while leaving his patient alone, or when his attention wanders and the patient wakes up enough to cough at a critical stage in the operation, or he fails to keep up with changes in vital signs, then he is worse than nothing. Such behavior can and does lead to cardiac arrest under anesthesia. Don't think it didn't happen in the early days when competition was scant or nonexistent. It still happens, though not as often.

Modern general anesthesia involves the uses of gases and intravenous agents. In addition to the anesthetic agents themselves, a number of drugs are used to paralyze skeletal muscle. This last group had its origin in jungle pharmacology, specifically curare used as arrow-tip poison in the Amazon forests. The drug relaxes muscles, thus requiring much less of the real anesthetic agents to control the patient during surgery, and allows the placing of a tube between the vocal cords and down toward the lungs to enhance breathing under anesthesia. But the drugs are dangerous; they paralyze breathing and require skilled use, and they do not relieve pain. A good anesthesiologist orchestrates this combination, with a minimum of toxic agents, to produce an optimal anesthetic state for the particular procedure to be done. Without question this person is a gift and blessing to modern life.

Beware of surgery in isolated places remote to the hospital, usually a doctor's office suite with a nurse anesthetist. A lot of cosmetic surgery is done this way. The surgeon might be the most attractive fellow, his results might be spectacular, and the anesthetist might be pretty and charming and competent, but suppose a really life-threatening complication happens. Then the backup of a fully equipped modern hospital will be needed with the authority of an anesthesiologist and readily available people who know how and can get to an arrested heart if they need to.

The remedy here depends upon the dedication of the anesthesiologist. So oriented he usually visits his patients before the surgery. Find out who this person is. The surgeons know; the house staff knows; the nurses in the operating room know; even the orderlies know. Beware of the hospital where the anesthesiologist retires to the doctor's lounge to laze around, usually fondling old magazines in a state of boredom, leaving the nurse in charge after induction of the anesthetic. Stay away from anesthesia and heavy sedation in doctor's offices, in dental offices, and in remote areas of the hospital. Deaths have occurred in dental chairs, during and after cosmetic surgery in offices, in MRI machines where no one can be in the tunnel with a child to watch for complications. Instances under these circumstances may seem to be sporadic, but a search reveals the problem to be commonplace (See Google, et al.). Complacency can be fatal.

Gases

Oxygen, carbon dioxide, nitrogen, compressed air, helium, nitrous oxide, and certain gaseous anesthetic agents are common in a hospital. Those used in treatment of patients are medical grade and are considered to be prescription drugs. Compressed gases also come in industrial grade, but this group should never be used medically. Some gases are used to power devices such as drills. Deaths and injuries have been reported from medical gas mix-ups. Connectors are designed to prevent confusion, and a mistake such as substituting carbon dioxide for oxygen, is impossible on wall supplies in the modern hospital unless someone changes connectors. Usually, only oxygen will be brought into a patient's room.

Trouble is Virtually eliminated in this arena if someone on the scene checks carefully to be sure the tank is, in fact, labeled as medical-grade oxygen. Oxygen creates a fire hazard, and neither visitors nor patients should smoke in its presence. Confused patients will try to smoke, even in an oxygen tent, if not carefully watched.

Chapter Eight
BLOOD TRANSFUSIONS

The risk of a blood transfusion is justified only if the patient's life depends upon it. Shock or near shock from life-threatening blood loss requires a transfusion without delay. Medically untreatable anemia may demand an ultimate resort to transfusion after a conservative approach to the problem has failed. The basics, the principles of the four blood types and the science of cross matching, are common knowledge. The patient must receive the correct blood type. Most blood transfusion errors occur from the patient's getting the wrong blood type. Even during the process of setting up a blood transfusion, a person trusts the labeling on the container of blood as it comes from the laboratory.

Unless the patient's life depends on rapid infusion of blood, the drip rate should be slow, and whatever the rate, a vigilant watch should be maintained for signs of trouble. Reaction may begin quite soon after only a small quantity of incompatible blood has entered the vein, five to 10 ml (equal to less than one teaspoon to one tablespoon). Apprehension, a feeling of something being wrong, agitation, flushing of the skin, and pain in the infusion vein, as well as abdominal, chest, or flank pain may appear. Even the slightest change is enough to justify shutting off the fluid flow and calling for medical help.

More delayed reactions include itching, hives (urticaria), fever, or any other changes in normal (usual) feelings and appearance.

The mechanisms of immediate reactions fall into several categories. The most frequent, acute hemolytic (destruction of red cells) transfusion reaction, carries the greatest immediate risk. Bacterially contaminated blood causes a sharp drop in blood pressure, shock, and chills. Acute lung injury due to transfusion causes coughing and trouble breathing. Severe allergic reactions cause breathing problems, chest and abdominal pain, and nausea. Again, any change in the patient after the transfusion has been started calls for the immediate stopping of the blood flow and reevaluation.

Delayed allergic and sensitivity reactions can occur. All the ramifications together constitute a highly complicated and specialized field, and immediate bedside intervention has little to do with prevention of later and secondary trouble. Delayed complications include the transmission of disease. In addition to bacterial infections, these include HIV, a leukemia virus, several hepatitis viruses, syphilis, malaria, Creutzfeldt-Jacob (a prion disease), and other infections and infestations carried in donor blood.

Blood for transfusions and the preparation of blood components in the United States comes largely from volunteer donors. The supply is chronically short, and the resources not always the most desirable. Strange indeed is the social demand for free blood. Why should the single most priceless and precious commodity on earth be given away by the donor, while the processors make money from it? When oil was worth $13 a barrel, the same amount of blood would have been worth $20,000 whole, or $67,000 processed. In 1998, the worldwide revenues from plasma-derived therapeutic products amounted to approximately a five-billion-dollar-a-year business (***Science Magazine***, March 15, 2003). The industry has continued to grow, and this could be a thriving endeavor using professional donors with a known clean health record. The current voluntary, allegedly altruistic, charity approach is not satisfactory.

To diminish any particular patient's risk, blood can be recovered during clean surgery (as in heart surgery), processed in the operating room, and transfused back into the patient if needed. A relative with compatible typing can give blood specifically for a particular patient, but this does not necessarily diminish the rate of infections such as hepatitis. Blood from parent to child may carry increased risk of immunological complications and consequent transfusion reactions.

Vigilance goes a long way in preventing disasters with transfusions. When a life depends upon a transfusion of blood or blood components in this complicated specialty, a patient or guardian can hardly do more than make sure the labels are right and be vigilant for early signs of a reaction. Someone needs to stay with the patient. The blood type on the label should match the patient's known blood type, and the name of the intended patient on the label should be identical to the name of the patient receiving the blood.

The patient's family might also try recruiting a clean healthy donor from among friends, or even pay for a healthy donor.

Chapter Nine
INFECTIONS

Down through the ages, millions of people died from ordinary infections, and the toll mounted sporadically as epidemics, plagues, and pestilence swept through Europe, Asia, and other countries, sometimes reducing the population by more than 40 percent. Waves of terror seized and panicked people in the wake of these disasters. Modern public health measures have eradicated most sources of scourges such as bubonic plague, anthrax, smallpox, and cholera, with only an occasional and limited outbreak occurring in scattered areas of the world's population. Malaria remains a problem in several countries.

Varro in 36 BC warned against living near swamps because they bred minute creatures "… which cannot be seen by the eyes, which float in the air and enter the body through the mouth and nose and there cause serious diseases." (Varro On Agriculture I, xii Loeb—via Google). Despite this ancient and startling insight, further development would be delayed some two thousand years, the cause of these disasters remaining a mystery to mankind until germs were discovered in the mid-nineteenth century. Then, truly effective agents against infections did not appear for another 70 years. So, just what is a germ? The term has become muddled from overuse. A fresh look in the Dictionary helps to bring back reality: Webster defines it as "A microorganism causing disease." Microorganism means you can't see the organism without the microscope or other magnification. And there is no old adage more characteristic of human thinking than this one: "Out of sight, out of mind," so the threat even today is too often ignored.

Here in the early twenty-first century, no one younger than 60 can even imagine the human predicament when no drugs were available to fight any one of the hundreds of deadly microorganisms. Death in ages gone by was commonplace from infections now easily controlled. Penicillin was discovered, in fact rediscovered, about 1930, yet its clinical application was delayed another 10 years. With this start, the antibiotic era developed during the remainder of the twentieth century, and continues to evolve. Before the era of antibiotics, infected flesh-and-bone injuries, pneumonia, meningitis, gangrene, gonorrhea, syphilis, peritonitis, diphtheria, typhoid fever, dysentery, and others ran a course determined only by the victim's innate body defenses.

Although antibiotics changed the grim realities of uncontrollable infections, they are not effective against all strains of infective agents, particularly certain causes of pneumonia, meningitis, wound infections, and others. Existing drugs have saved millions of lives, but infection remains the major destroyer of life. Many infections and deaths are preventable, and too many are related to the hospital environment. Such disasters have been occurring for a long time and probably gave rise to the term, "pest house," or the even more damning, "pest hole." Doubtless, such complications are as old as the first hospital. Until the discovery of microorganisms (bacteria in this instance) mankind was totally blind to this invisible and deadly enemy.

As an example of such tragic dilemmas, in mid-nineteenth century Vienna, a conscientious Hungarian obstetrician named Ignatz Semmelweiss wondered why the most exclusive women's ward carried a high mortality rate from childbed fever (puerperal sepsis), despite being attended by the best trained doctors of the time, and eager, intelligent medical students. The rate had risen to more than 20 percent, while at the same time, the mortality rate remained at less than four percent in another ward down the hall, attended by midwives only. In pondering the problem he wondered if the doctors were the cause. And so it proved to be.

Semmelweiss guessed right after the death of a pathologist friend who nicked his finger while doing an autopsy on a victim of childbed fever, and then quickly died with symptoms of childbed fever. The doctors were spreading the cause of the fatal illness by doing something wrong. At the time, germs had never been named; sterile technique was unheard of; antibiotics were beyond the doctors' wildest dreams, and nobody understood the real nature of infection. They spouted such nonsense as "laudable pus." Doctors and students, wearing their street clothes, were going directly from the autopsy room, after dissecting the bodies of childbed fever victims, to the bedside. There they examined mothers and delivered babies without first washing their hands. The contaminated hands were carrying the invisible cause directly to the mothers. Semmelweiss said so, and set up a regimen of hand washing.

The arrogant medical mentality reacted violently. Doctors killing their own patients! Doctors spreading the disease! Doctors having to wash their hands! The very idea was decried as nonsense, and Semmelweiss labeled as crazy. They turned against him. He lost his practice and was driven out of Vienna. This happened in the days before Lister and Pasteur, before germs were recognized as the cause of infections. But the fate of Semmelweiss reflects the mindset of the pack. Only years later did compulsory hand washing become a requirement for surgeons, obstetricians, and others.

Yet, the lack of hand washing remains a problem in the modern hospital, and the lack of its being done and done properly is still a major cause of hospital-acquired (nosocomial) infections. Current studies reveal this: strict observance of the hand-washing rule would eliminate a large percentage of hospital infections, but it has not happened yet. Stubbornness, forgetfulness, negligence of medical personnel, failure to take precautions seriously, and the invisibility of germs keep the germs in business.

Human behavior does not change essentially in a mere 160 years. There have always been fads in the practice of medicine, and fads will continue. There will always be the thing to do for a particular problem at a particular time, and any person, doctor or otherwise, who discovers and reveals the fallacy of such thinking will meet with resistance and ridicule. Think of phlebotomy, or venesection. The attending doctors bled George Washington severely and repeatedly as he was dying from pneumonia. The treatment only weakened his already weak condition. But medical opinion considered it to be the proper treatment, at a time when no effective treatment for pneumonia existed. Survival depended upon the patient's natural defense mechanisms, and certainly not upon what the doctor knew to do. If George Washington had died without being bled, someone no doubt would have blamed the doctor for not doing the bleeding procedures, and in the modern temperament he might have been sued for malpractice.

Carelessness and ignorance about germs continues into the twenty-first century, and many hospital complications, neartragedies, and deaths are due directly to this fault. Here is a real example of its treachery. Mrs. Steven Downy arrived at her brother Robert's hospital room to find him in a mess, lying on his side, grasping the lifted side rail. She was astonished. He had been improving beyond hopes of the family, and she had come to take him home. "Robert, what's wrong?" she asked.

"I'm bleeding," he said. "Just look at my bed. I'm over here trying to keep out of the blood." She looked. The sheets were bloody, and the blood had formed a puddle in the bed and on the floor. She searched for the cause and found it—the subclavian line. The nurse had removed the line according to doctor's orders, applied a dressing and left him alone. Blood dribbled down from the beneath the blood-soaked dressing and trickled over Robert's chest wall. His face, body and hands were smeared red. Mrs. Downy stormed out of the room and down to the nurses' station, and found the errant nurse. They returned to the room in a hurry. The nurse donned sterile gloves and changed the dressing, using a larger bandage and more pressure to stop the bleeding.

Did the nurse change gloves after removing the bloody dressing with her fingers? No, as Mrs. Downy told it later, wearing the same gloves, she popped open a pack of gauze, grasped the new dressing in her fingers, applied it to the bleeding wound, then taped it tightly and didn't clean the surrounding skin with a disinfectant.

Robert had made a dramatic improvement from the symptoms of an obscure blood abnormality, too much of the wrong protein. He had undergone a six-stage plasma exchange, through the indwelling catheter in his subclavian vein. All of his blood had been removed in increments, the blood cells separated from the plasma and returned to the patient along with six big doses of human albumin.

The crippling symptoms of the disease had improved to an encouraging degree.

With the bleeding staunched at the needle puncture site, Robert seemed to be no worse for the experience. The nurses discharged him, and Mrs. Downy took him to her home. The family celebrated the medical triumph at dinner the same evening.

The next morning, Robert failed to respond to his sister's knock on the bedroom door and her cheery, "Breakfast's ready." She entered the room. Robert lay drawn up in a knot, covered in sweat, and shaking with chills. She palmed his forehead. He was burning with fever and too delirious to answer her questions. The rescue squad rushed him to the emergency room. "Hospital-induced staphylococcus infection causing a virulent septicemia (bloodstream infection)," were the angry and anguished words of the emergency room doctor. The puncture wound where the catheter had been used and later removed was swollen and inflamed. Robert improved with massive doses of antibiotics fed through another indwelling catheter over a period of 10 days. Robert survived, but his old symptoms returned, worse than ever.

Most likely, the infection came from one or more breaks in technique, the worst when the nurse changed the bloody bandage. Once a sterile glove touches an unsterile object, it is contaminated, and the germs are passed on, in this case to the gauze she picked up with the contaminated glove and applied to the open wound.

As later investigation revealed, when she removed the catheter she did not use an antiseptic on the surrounding skin before clipping the one holding stitch and sliding the catheter out. As we know from the ensuing complications, the hole through the skin and vein wall remained open, and blood ran out on the skin. No doubt certain germs in the surrounding skin flora entered the opening. Of course, there are other possibilities, too many to be controlled entirely.

Adherence to proper precautions and technique go furthest in preventing most hospital-acquired infections. But the problem is far more serious than either the public or the medical profession generally recognizes. Everyone knows the danger of infection is lurking, but to average thinking, such an oddity is not likely to happen. People simply expect to go into the hospital and get prescribed treatments or planned surgery and come out unscathed.

For the sobering facts, pull up Google or another Internet search engine, and type in "hospital infections." The numbers are astonishing: a hundred thousand or more deaths per year, more than twice the death rate from traffic accidents in United States. The cost is in the billions of dollars for the more than two million infections picked up by hospitalized patients. These infections from a variety of germs occur in any organ system and arise from two sources. Most are due to contamination of one sort or another in the hospital environment, but some are due to germs harbored in or on the patient's body until illness weakens the normal resistance, and the enemy begins to take over.

Indwelling urinary catheters and ventilation tubes carry an increased risk of infection, each with its own particular flora. Proper technique at the time of insertion will decrease the danger of infection. The subclavian line invites infection in the surrounding soft tissue and the bloodstream. The most scrupulous sterile technique should be used during the insertion, but this procedure most of the time is done in an ICU, and the setting leaves something to be desired in the way of optimum protection against infection.

A second source of infection lurks in and on the human body at all times. These attacks are more difficult to prevent and treat, and some present with deadly treachery, as happened to another unfortunate patient, poor Archie Duke. No one understood the increasing pain in his right thigh, and various doctors and nurses and others made guesses when his family brought him to the emergency room repeatedly as his symptoms grew more intense. Their guesses included "psychological." Archie held all kinds of promise. He was 16 years old, good-looking, good student, well behaved, and the high school's best football player. He had a cute girl friend, a zest for life, and he planned to go to college in two years. At afternoon scrimmage, he had been butted mid-thigh by the helmeted head of another player. Pain became progressively more intense at the site of impact. He stayed in the game until practice ended, but the pain grew. The team doctor sent him home with ice packs. He was in the emergency room several times before midnight with increasing pain in the thigh, and Archie Duke was dead within three days.

The impact with the helmet bruised a deep thigh muscle, and the muscle began to swell. Archie developed what is known as **compartment syndrome**, but it went unrecognized. The muscle, confined and trapped within its barriers, its own surrounding bone, ligaments and fascia, continued to swell until it compressed and finally blocked its own blood and nerve supply. The initially bruised muscle died, and as swelling increased, more muscle died.

The lurking bacterial flora of the body, unfortunately, this time the deadly streptococcus, invaded the dead muscle and multiplied rapidly. Archie developed a fever, but it did not make sense to the doctors who saw him. The skin had not been broken, and the infection could not be related to the injury, so they thought. When the thigh became swollen and hard and peculiar-looking, a general surgeon was called. He too was unfamiliar with compartment syndrome, but he did open the thigh and take out some dead muscle, but by then Archie had full-blown septic shock, and the flesh-eating bacteria had progressed further upward.

Finally, a plastic surgeon trained in major reconstructive procedures was called into consultation. He recognized the illness, and at the family's urging did the only thing left to try, a hemi-pelvectomy (the highest amputation possible, including part of the body). But too late, the bacterial destruction already had progressed beyond even these limits, and Archie died. Had this last surgeon been called on the night after the injury, a simple opening of the fascia confining the muscle, would have released the pressure and stopped the muscle destruction and subsequent fatal infection.

One of the most feared infections in modern times is due to the so-called flesh-eating bacteria, a strain of streptococcus pyogenes, or Group A streptococcus. This particular germ is responsible for several diseases, among them strep throat, scarlet fever, purulent skin and underlying tissue infections, necrotizing (dead tissue) fascitis, the flesh-eating disease also called streptococcal gangrene, and streptococcal toxic shock syndrome (STSS), which carries a high mortality rate. The last three can occur in deadly progression. Some survivors remain crippled by rheumatic fever, kidney damage, and other complications. The infection can begin at the site of a deep hidden injury, with no immediate involvement of the skin, or it can begin with a minor skin injury.

Minor open wounds, appearing not to be worth a trip to the emergency room, should be washed with soapy water, followed by rinsing under the flowing tap, then the application of temporary pressure and drying with a clean paper towel, and finally the application of a sterile dressing. Triple antibiotic ointment may dispatch lurking organisms and help salve your worries. Several companies are now selling small sterile dressings containing antibiotics. Caustic, burning, alcohol, iodine, and Merthiolate types of antiseptics are unnecessary and may do more harm than good by damaging the exposed tissue in the wound.

Archie's tragedy falls in a category of a treatable disease being bungled to a fatal outcome. Here is yet another, also involving a teenage boy. James was an exceptional scholar with great promise, who unfortunately, had been was born with a breastbone (sternum) deformity. Following elective and corrective surgery on a Friday morning, James showed a deficient production of urine but received a pain medication known for serious side effects. During the weekend following surgery, James became progressively sicker, with increasing belly pain and swelling. The nurses and residents were dismissive of the mother's concerns, labeled the symptoms as being due to gas, and told the family nothing could be done about gas, this being a colossal bit of misinformation. As James became progressively sicker, the hospital personnel chose to ignore the mother's requests for a senior doctor to be called in. The operating surgeon had gone away for the weekend. The boy died early Monday afternoon from shock and sepsis due to a ruptured ulcer in the digestive track. This was a preventable death, caused by unrecognized complications of a dangerous drug accumulating to toxic levels in the absence of normal kidney function.

Here again is the mindset. They put a handle (title) on a situation and defended the error to the death. A handle, a name, a label can be dismissive but is never a real understanding or explanation and certainly not appropriate treatment. What is a family to do when caught in a situation like this one? The mother tried, but no one listened. The hospital personnel paved the boy's path to death with pat explanations. The answer simply is this: When the intimidating atmosphere created by the attitude of hospital personnel fails to bluff the family, then something can be done in these circumstances. Someone has to wake up and take over. Go to a telephone and call the surgeon himself. If he is away, another senior surgeon will be covering his calls. Get him. If this doesn't work, call the family doctor, the doctor who referred the patient to the surgeon. Go down to the hospital administrator's office. Someone will be there even on weekends. Bring the problem to administration's attention in firm but polite terms. Demand medical intervention. Go to the head nurses' office. Someone is always there. Or call your lawyer as a last resort.

But how in this world of modern medicine is a family, all laymen, to know enough to confront the establishment set stubbornly on the road to a terrible mistake? The answer lies in the ability to admit something is not under control and a determination to act on this insight. These two unfortunate patients, Archie and James, were caught in a progressive and deadly dilemma. So, when should a family use any tactic necessary to intercede and come to the rescue of the victim? The answer: **When something new and threatening to their lives is happening** and getting progressively worse. This is the principle for every concerned person to follow; a new set of symptoms complicating an illness or injury or appearing out of the blue is reason for concern, then alarm. When these symptoms progressively worsen, then it is time for immediate expert medical intervention.

Beware of weekends. Don't go into a hospital for an elective major operation unless the operating surgeon plans to be there for the post-operative care. He may operate on Friday and go out of town for the weekend, leaving his partner or a colleague in charge, but it is not quite the same. The substitute does not have a feel for the case where he did not do the surgery, and he may be reluctant to treat another doctor's patient, and, consequently, he may hesitate dangerously. Nobody is happy to be working on the weekend; they just want to get through it, and they are likely to be overloaded with only a skeletal crew. It is not the time to get the best attention, especially should the need for attention become desperate.

But more about infections–The Center for Disease Control and Prevention has awarded research grants to eight epicenters, including Johns Hopkins and Harvard, to find ways to improve control over microorganisms. The best medical magazines, among them the **New England Journal of Medicine, Annals of Internal Medicine, Journal of the American College of Surgeons,** and **Journal of the American Medical Association,** are addressing the problems of infection. Lay periodicals have been established for this sole purpose, and numerous books by journalists and physicians have been published on the subject. The Institute of Medicine of the National Academy of Science has issued its alarming report, and major industry is behind efforts of the Leapfrog Group to eliminate medical errors. The major medical societies all have begun to wrestle with the problem of patient safety. The Internet furnishes an almost endless supply of information on this subject.

The remedy for much of this trouble is readily available. The source of infection, as every grammar school student knows, remains always invisible to the naked eye. "If you can't see it, it can't hurt you," seems to be the incautious assumption. In this invisible world, the number of living organisms on the skin of each person varies from count to count, one report stating it to be larger than the total population of all human beings living on the planet. Carelessness with this waiting treachery and short cuts transmit many hospital-acquired infections. Every vulnerable person should watch the doctors and the nurses. Each of them by training and by the rules must ALWAYS wash hands with soap and water or a sterilizing solution before and after touching a patient. The doctor who goes from one patient to the next without washing carries germs from one to the other. If he goes all day or all afternoon without washing, he is carrying quite a load. By the end of the day he doubtless has become deadly. Only a person's immune system will keep him from becoming sick from the doctor's touch.

Does the doctor come in the room, stand by the bedside and thumb through the chart, shake hands with one or more visitors, put his hands on the bed rail, then examine his patient without first going to the sink and washing? Does he go to the sink and wash after he touches the patient? If he does neither, then the patient has a problem and so do the rest of his patients. And the nurse, and those who rank beneath her, the one wearing the gloves—is she wearing the gloves to protect herself or to protect the patient? If she puts them on new just for the patient, adheres to strict sterile technique, and discards them when through, then she wears them to protect the patient. If she wears the same pair from one patient to another, then she is wearing them for a reason she herself does not understand, like a false sense of security. Contaminated gloves, like the unwashed hand, can carry germs too. If the nurse enters the room wearing a pair of so-called sterile gloves and approaches the patient's bed without changing them, look out. Don't let her do it. She is careless or ignorant or both, and dangerous.

When the doctor appears, a stethoscope very likely will be hanging around his neck. After a bit of preliminary, he puts the ear-pieces in his ears and with one hand lifts the bell end toward the skin of a chest. It's going to be icy cold, everyone knows; it hasn't failed yet. But of greater seriousness, when did he last clean with alcohol or soap and water the rims of the business end of this magnificent symbol of medicine? How about never? And it has been applied to some exotic places. Call him on it.

Another disguised threat usually wears a white coat. Notice the safety pin fastened in the front lapel. He's usually a neurology type or the man who has to do a complete physical. The pin is for testing pain perception, and for scratching the sole of a foot to see if the toes rebel in the right direction (Babinski toe sign, they call it). Chances are this one little pin has done a lot of traveling. The doctor has pecked and scratched the skin of everyone he has examined. Pain perception sometimes needs to be tested in remote and sensuous areas of the body where the more lush bacterial habitation is likely to be flourishing. Has he had the pin one day or five years? Does he sterilize it after each patient? Is he the rough type who draws blood every time he pecks the skin to test pain perception? Does he get a new pin for each patient?

The pin can spread and transmit everyday staphylococci and other unexotic pests. Prion diseases can be transmitted this way, the most notorious being Creutzfeldt-Jacob disease (similar to mad-cow disease), a relentless non-treatable invasion progressively destroying the brain until the brain resembles a sponge, thus the other name, spongiform encephalopathy. Ordinary sterilization does not kill the responsible agent. Soaking a contaminated instrument in strong bleach is believed to be effective. Has he soaked his pin in bleach? Call him on it. This group of diseases is infrequent in humans, but small chance does not justify the risk.

A variation on the same theme, this fellow wears a white coat, too, but carries no safety pin. He has something fancier, a bright stainless steel pinwheel with a handle about six inches long, riding in his breast pocket. It serves the same purpose as the safety pin, but has the appearance of being in a bit higher class. Does he wash it after each patient? Has it ever been near bleach, soap and water, or alcohol? If not, don't let him use it.

The problem with infections across the entire spectrum of medicine even in modern times remains too complicated with too many ramifications for any one person to control. What can the patient do to guard himself, other than caring for his own personal hygiene and choosing his doctor and hospital carefully? Neither patients nor hospital personnel like the unavoidable answer to this question. For a beginning, quite simply call nurse and doctor alike on sloppy technique, and if not sure, raise the question anyway. It will make them pause to think. Ignore the hostile reaction. It's being done to patients, not to them. In these circumstances in the modern medical jungle, only vigilance will save the defenseless. But the hand-washing fault is only a part of the picture; infections can and do come by other avenues.

The problem remains too big for everyone concerned, as is evident by the scientific, social, and commercial efforts now being made to improve patient safety and to remedy the damage being done by the system, including infections and other hospital complications.

According to estimates from the Centers for Disease Control and Prevention (CDC), about two million patients in the United States each year pick up infections while hospitalized for other causes, at a cost of nearly five billion dollars for treatment, and of these about 90,000 die from the infections. Infections also occur in clinics, dialysis units, nursing homes, and other long-term care facilities. CDC officials consider clean hands to be the most important method of controlling the spread of infection (germs). Alcohol-based hand lotions are recommended for cleaning and disinfecting the hands. You can buy this product in any drugstore or supermarket, or you can buy your own glycerin and rubbing alcohol and mix the two to suit your own sense of touch. Play safe and buy the ready-made product, but just plain rubbing alcohol will kill most of the germs on hands. Nosocomial (hospital-acquired) bloodstream infections, according to CDC, are the eighth leading cause of death in the United States. Seventy percent of these occur to patients with central venous catheters.

This grim situation has not changed, even today, the figures about the same, as reported in the New York Times Sunday October 28, 2007, describing over 19,000 deaths from methicillin-resistant staphylococcus aureus (MRSA), and upward of a total of 99,000 deaths from hospital-acquired infections in the period of one year. The New Yorker magazine, August 11 & 18, 2008 under the title, SUPERBUGS describes the growing spread, the growing resistance, and the growing death rate in hospitals from bacteria such as the gram-negative Klebsiella, the MRSA, certain strains of E. Coli, and others.

One authority reported a 90 percent reduction in this infection rate by the use of antibiotic-bonded catheters (minocycline and Rifampin). All of this information can be studied in detail at the Joint Commission on Accreditation of Healthcare Organizations' Web site (***www.jcaho.org***).

Chapter Ten
X-RAY

The hospital radiologist is a doctor who looks at X-ray pictures of various parts of the human body then records a report of what he sees. He talks about a picture, not a patient. This information is computerized, or a secretary types those words, and the report is put in the patient's record in the hospital, or mailed to the office of the doctor who sent the patient to the X-ray department for outpatient pictures; he did not refer the patient to the radiologist. The general radiologist has no patients. Members of the X-ray department staff, mostly technicians, make the pictures on various areas of people sent to the X-ray department by other doctors. Ordinarily, the radiologist has contact with patients only for special studies like the gastrointestinal (GI) series and the barium enema. He helps make the pictures during these examinations.

To give radiology its just due, in recent years, the interventionist radiologist has evolved. He punctures arteries, guides wires, catheters, and coils up the blood vessels for various purposes, and places stents to lessen partial obstructions in various arteries. Most of this work is precarious, and a surgeon should be readily available as a precaution should real trouble develop. The CAT scan, the MRI, and radiation therapy have stimulated specialization in those particular branches housed by radiology. Certain radiologists have become radiation oncologists and are in the department during working hours to supervise treatments.

However, the general radiologist does not see most of the patients who come to the X-ray department for studies. He puts the pictures up on a view box, looks at them, and dictates. This is good enough when he sees a problem correctly and records it correctly. But with one picture after another popping up to be read, it is entirely impersonal and too easy for the man doing the dictating not to recognize the damage careless words can do.

Several games go on here. They have to do mainly with the plaintiff's lawyer (malpractice), and the IRS (income taxes), or perhaps just not knowing when to shut up. To protect himself against being sued for misreading X-ray pictures, the radiologist names several possibilities imaginable at the moment. Then he may suggest a certain diagnostic procedure as follow-through, or even a certain treatment. In the meantime the patient might have gone back home to as far as the other coast of the United States, or the patient already might have undergone surgery, or embarked on a course of treatment. The diagnostic procedure recommended could be outmoded, uncalled for, or sometimes correct. The radiologist's guesswork almost never measures up to the judgment of the specialist who sent the patient to the X-ray department for studies. On the other hand, some doctors, especially those with less training, are naïve enough to accept the radiologist's language as gospel and proceed to follow the suggestions.

Where do the radiologist's recommendations put the patient's doctor? Occasionally, the suggestions may help, but usually they put the doctor in charge out on a limb. If something adverse happens, a plaintiff's attorney can twist the circumstances on the radiologist's spurious recommendations, and accuse the patient's doctor of not practicing up to standards. Other doctors refer to this habit among radiologists as "covering your ass."

An unnecessary statement at the end of the radiologist's report says, "Thank you for referring this patient." This statement substantiates the radiologist's claim to being in the private practice of medicine, when he actually is an employee of the hospital. It makes a difference in the tax write-offs.

At night in emergency cases, the orthopedic surgeon, neurosurgeon, general surgeon, and others read the X-ray pictures made on their patients by the technicians on call. They come to a decision about treatment and proceed with a necessary emergency operation. The radiologist sees the pictures the next day, dictates a report, and charges the patient.

Every conscientious and careful doctor visits the X-ray department to see the X-ray pictures of his hospitalized patients and study them with a radiologist. He never takes a radiologist's word without checking the pictures himself. This makes for good collaboration in the diagnostic process. It helps to prevent both doctors from misreading the films. A good radiologist has to be a smart person, well versed in the principles of medicine, and very careful about what he says and does.

Radiologists can and do make crashing errors. Here is an example. A young surgical resident in a Midwestern hospital got sick enough to be a patient in his own hospital, a simple case of the flu but with a fever of 103 degrees. As part of the evaluation a chest X-ray picture was made to rule out pneumonia. The next day, the radiologist sent word to the doctor saying they had found a lesion, which might be tuberculosis and to be sure to have another chest X-ray picture in a month for follow up. The sick doctor shot out of bed, fever and all, and raced down to the X-ray department. He checked out his own film jacket and approached the radiologist, who sat in a director's chair with the words Dr. Edwards (not his real name) in big black letters across the white canvas back. The doctor snapped his chest picture on the view box and asked the radiologist to show him the lesion. A small round chalky area was pointed out. The patient reached up and with one swipe of his forefinger removed the lesion, a splatter of developing fluid on the film. This was one of the quickest cures on record of active tuberculosis.

Imagine the callousness, this chief of a department doing such a frightening and unconcerned thing to a young person. Something like it could happen to anyone. A patient should not accept recommendations or damaging news coming out of an X-ray department until the findings have been rechecked thoroughly. Get the X-ray films and another opinion to find out whether a suggested course of action is really necessary.

There are direct dangers to a patient in an X-ray department. The patient can fall or be dropped off a table. Some examinations call for the table to be tilted up and down in the dark. Allergic reaction to an injected dye or to medications given by mouth can create a sudden crisis. The puncture sites in arteries can bleed to the point of requiring surgical repair. Fatal hemorrhage has occurred at the site of femoral artery puncture. During an interventionist procedure any number of things can go wrong, some requiring immediate surgery. In X-ray therapy, patients and dosage should be checked carefully. A tumor-killing dose of radiation certainly should not be given to the wrong patient or to the wrong site in the right patient. Nor should the patient be given an accidental overdose.

The single most important non X-ray machine, the MRI equipment, is hazardous to any patient with ferromagnetic metal in the body anywhere. The magnetic field of this machine is powerful enough to cause hairpins and safety pins to fly about, and to move larger pieces of ferromagnetic metal buried anywhere in the patient. Such ferromagnetic metal is usually stainless steel, like certain orthopedic splints, aneurysm clips of 1960s vintage in the skull cavity, wire sutures, and some joint replacements.

Recently, a national television network aired the story of a woman in whose abdomen a very large surgical instrument had been left, but this is not so uncommon. The method for investigating the possibility requires caution. In past years, almost all surgical instruments for cutting and clamping and retracting have been made of a highly ferromagnetic type of stainless steel. Accidentally leaving them in an abdominal or chest wound no doubt will continue to happen. It is important in post-operative surgical patients with complications to have a plain X-ray picture of the surgical area before resorting to MRI. Inside a body cavity, movement of a surgical instrument in the magnetic field could be very damaging if not fatal.

Here is another X-ray disgrace. A middle-aged English immigrant, Greta Hudson, worked as a cocktail waitress in a renowned western ski resort. She made her living serving drinks and in her spare time, skied and hiked and snow-shoed, and looked after her health and kept to a regular exercise regimen. Her mammograms had been negative every year, and she was thankful. Then one year, her fifth for an annual mammogram, a new radiologist saw a lesion. The resultant breast biopsy identified a malignant growth. She had many well-to-do friends in the resort, and they took her to a center where radical surgery found invasive cancer already invading lymph nodes of the axilla (armpit). After chemotherapy and radiation treatments, all her hair fell out and she wore a wig over her bald scalp while the hair re-grew.

The doctor who performed her surgery sent for the old mammograms. The very first one showed the growth in an earlier stage, and others showed it slowly enlarging in the breast. The radiologist reading the films had missed the lesion every year. Theoretically, removal of the growth five years earlier would have made a difference in Greta's hopes for long-term survival. She confronted her doctor, the one who has taken care of her everyday needs for years, and who referred her for mammograms. He had never looked at the pictures himself. He had simply trusted the radiological report. Frightened, depressed, sad, frustrated, confused, defeated – a peaceful soul, she sued no one. She died three years later from widespread metastases of the breast cancer. .

These warnings lead back to the patient. Every adverse X-ray report should be checked and double-checked for errors, especially errors in labeling. Every X-ray picture should be checked for correct interpretation. Pictures made of patients with multiple injuries should be checked for missed fractures and bleeding. When a patient or a member of the patient's family receives bad news based upon an X-ray finding, someone should ask to see the pictures with the radiologist. Ask him to point out the abnormality. Double-check the identification. Check the pathology reported by the radiologist. Remember, these men do not practice medicine, they make pictures and they ***practice pictures***. Pictures made during screening studies, mammograms and colonoscopies for deadly malignancies should be double- and triple-checked for missed lesions, correct labeling, and false positive readings.

Chapter Eleven
PLASTIC SURGERY

A well-trained and ethical plastic surgeon contributes enormously to improving the human condition. Cleft lips, cleft palates, and other birth defects and deformities, the depressing ravages of old age (quivering wattles hanging from old chins), motion problems of crippled limbs, severe skin damage from burns, the terrible deformities of injuries, and other debilitating problems are greatly mended by his expertise.

Well-trained means he has completed a required course in general surgery, then has completed a residency in plastic surgery. Many plastic surgeons go on with further training to specialize in a narrow sub-specialty such as hand surgery or advanced reconstructive techniques. Some confine their work to cosmetic surgery of the face and neck, and the good results make many people happy and improve the quality of their lives. When a town gets its first competent plastic surgeon, his beautiful work becomes the envy of established surgeons not trained in his refined techniques. His skin scars are almost invisible.

Despite the good these doctors can do, the patient cannot afford to be careless in choosing because no field of conventional medicine is more fraught with quacks, frauds, and the inept. One of them can ruin a person in a minute. Those of this stripe, pretending to be plastic surgeons, tend to settle in communities of old retired people with money, and they advertise. They do operations on face, breast, and body in private offices away from hospital premises. This is a dangerous business at best. Some are not doctors of medicine, or doctors of anything. Others have no formal training in plastic surgery. Vanity and limited funds can cause an unhappy person to be fooled into taking a risk with a surgeon who charges less and is not competent. The results can vary from disfiguration to death. Also, faces are ruined even in the hands of a trained person who just does it wrong, for instance, the late middle-aged woman whose face is as slick and shiny as a peeled onion, her eye sockets sunken, her expression hollow-eyed and gaunt, from overzealous surgery.

Short cuts are dangerous. The injection of various chemicals like botox carries its own inherent risk, and if done at all, it should be in the hands of a specialist trained to do this work. The laser is not a magic wand. It is an instrument of destruction, like the knife. When used correctly it does the intended job, but it can be more dangerous than the knife. When used the wrong way it can cook deep. The scarring and disfigurement is permanent and worse than the reasons for the initial surgery. This instrument does not belong in the hands of the untrained. For cosmetic work, it serves only as an addition to the equipment used by a competent plastic surgeon.

An ethical doctor will not operate on someone just because the person wants, or thinks she wants it done. He should be aware of mental and psychological problems manifested as fixations on an imagined physical blemish or defect. He should help the patient get the real guidance she needs. The extreme form of such a fixation is known as Body Dysmorphic Disorder. It has to do with body image and is not a real defect. Surgery is not the treatment or the cure.

Some people need a word of encouragement and need to be told they look just fine the way they are. Converting a handsome aquiline nose into a cute little Hollywood stub can ruin the appearance of the rest of a person's face; the eyes may then appear to be too far apart in a dish-faced plateau. The plastic surgeon knows the fault, but the patient does not.

The main caution here—for elective cosmetic work, choose carefully. Find some of his patients. If they have slick faces and sunken eyes or everted eyelids, keep looking.

To take fewer chances, find a competent plastic surgeon who does his work in a hospital with an anesthesiologist for both sedation and deeper anesthesia. No one gets a second chance if something goes wrong in an office isolated from the hospital.

Several specialty fields overlap with plastic surgery. Ear, nose, and throat specialists perform radical neck dissections for cancer, especially when the growth arises in the larynx (voice box). Some of these specialists are formally trained for this surgery, but others are a bit out of their element. Traditionally this has been the territory of the general surgeon. The hardcore plastic surgeon has been taught how to do this deforming (deeply scarred neck, permanent opening in the trachea) and disabling (loss of normal voice) operation. Cases are likely to fall into his hands when the primary malignancy involves other neck areas or the head and face. Oral surgeons try to and sometimes do break into this field, and some dentists without advanced training call themselves oral surgeons. Few if any are qualified to do large surgical procedures on the face and neck. Some ophthalmologists (eye doctors) revise sagging eyelids, and a competent subspecialty has developed in this endeavor.

Dermatologists are getting into the very lucrative field of facial alterations with lasers, knives, and chemicals, some without previous formal training.

Self-trained, untrained, and outright charlatans are performing liposuction. This operation can be dangerous, even fatal and belongs in the hands of the qualified surgeon.

Breast enhancement has attracted a host of surgical frauds, and some of the resulting disasters have been well publicized. Cosmetic plastic surgery is never an emergency. There is ample time for caution.

Chapter Twelve
A VIEW FROM INSIDE

Listen to these extracts from the author's (A) interview with an experienced registered nurse (RN) employed by a teaching hospital in a major city with a first-rate medical school:

RN: "The nurse worked on this man for two hours, cleaned him up and with her dirty gloves, turned around and fiddled with the IV apparatus."

A: "What was the man's problem?"

RN: "He came in with a fractured hip. They did a total hip replacement, and he was elderly, had lost a lot of weight and was not mobile, and he messed the bed. So the nurse, the nurse's assistant, not the nurse, she came in and cleaned him up then started messing with his IV."

A: "With the same pair of gloves?

RN: "That's right. A few days later the man's son tells me his Dad's made a turn for the worst, he's septic (infected), and the doctors can't figure out where it came from, and I said, 'Where do you think it came from?' "

A: "Did the man die?"

RN: "Last time I checked, he was not mobile but still living. I tell you what's going on now. They hit him with vancomycin and Irvaquin, high-priced and high-powered antibiotics, whatever the drug rep had managed to sell the doctor that month. Until they find out what the infection is, the patient will stay on high-powered drugs that blast everything. The next time that old man needs an antibiotic, it won't be effective."

A: "A common practice?"

RN: "Yes, and the family members need to get them out of the hospital. Patients like the old man get antibiotic-resistant infections, like MRSA (methicillin-resistant staphylococcus aureus), or acinetobacter. They get that bug whenever they are on the ventilator for any length of time. There are all kinds of great new bugs. A patient will develop pneumonia because the nurses just let them lie there. On the weekends the nurse assistants will let them lie there for four hours. We have a lot of cases that come in with one thing and end up with pneumonia because they lie in the bed and don't move."

A: "On the weekends?"

RN: "Here was a typical weekend when I was a floor nurse. Nobody got a bath or their bed changed, and nobody got ice or water. When a meal came, the nurse assistant put it on a tray and left it on the little bedside table and walked off. If the patients couldn't feed themselves that was it."

A: "Who was in charge?"

RN: "The ones who needed to do something about it would never do anything about it. By Sunday night the floor stank real bad. There were only two nurses with 24 patients to feed, bathe, and medicate. It was more than anyone could handle. That's why I left the hospital system. I couldn't stand what they were doing to the poor patients."

A: "Tell me more."

RN: "This man was admitted, a diabetic, already a BKA on one side."

A: "What is a BKA?"

RB: "A below-the-knee amputee on one side. His symptoms were on the other leg. It was cool with no pulses, a lot of pain, and redness. The doctors brought in consultants, and the man sat there for three days while they tried to get a cardiac work-up, and preparing to do a fem-pop."

A: "Explain how a fem-pop works."

RN: "It's a graft, a bypass from the big artery in the thigh, the femoral artery, to a major branch further down in the lower leg, the popliteal artery. It's a last-ditch effort to save the foot and lower leg."

A: "Sounds desperate."

RN: "Anything to save the leg. Cardiology comes in and does a work-up, EKGs and the other tests. They say he's ready to go, but not the best candidate in the world. For two more days the surgeon, like he hasn't read the consultation notes, writes on the chart he's awaiting cardiac clearance. I told the charge nurse the patient had clearance. Why were we waiting? The patient had been in the hospital for three days, lying in his room with his leg getting colder. The charge nurse said it was up to the doctor, but she never approached the doctor to ask why he was waiting. The next day the cardiologist was doing rounds, and she was so angry, she pressed so hard with her ballpoint she nearly went through the paper. The cardiologist asked, 'I gave given this man cardiac clearance, what are we waiting for? He is going to lose his leg. Why wait any longer? His foot is turning blacker and colder. What is the holdup?'"

A: "What happened?"

RN: "They went in and did the fem-pop finally, but they had waited so long he ended up an AKA (above the knee amputee) on that side. He died the following Sunday."

A: "From what?"

RN: "Complication of diabetes."

A: "In the hospital?"

RN: "Yes, in and out of the hospital. He never recovered from the complications and the surgery."

A: "If someone had been demanding attention for this man, he may have had a chance. As it was, he slipped through the cracks."

RN: "I looked back over the chart. The cardiologist's handwriting was very clear, very legible."

A: "I take it problems like this were the rule, not the exception."

RN: "We had a PCA pump malfunction one time and kill a woman."

A: "What's a PCA pump?"

RN: "That's your pain pump, patient-controlled anesthesia. It's hooked into your IV, and the IV fluids have to run at 25cc or more."

A: "This is astounding."

RN: "The PCA is supposed to be set for either a continuous basal rate or for boluses, and they set it wrong. The pump malfunctioned, and it overdosed this woman on Dilaudid and killed her. She had come in for a total abdominal hysterectomy."

A: "What made it malfunction?

RN: "They don't know. Maybe a computer chip."

A: "Could the accident have been prevented?"

RN: "Had a nurse been in her room more often and noticed the woman was out of it, yes."

A: "If the family had been there and noticed she had passed out they could have stopped it."

RN: "A lot of times at night, the nurses won't go in the room for hours at a time."

A: "This didn't happen at a nursing home. It was in a hospital."

RN: "A hospital. I tried to read the documentation, and there was none. I hate this flow sheet charting they've gone to. No one fits into the cubbyhole of flow sheet charting. The nurses check off words like neuro, okay. People don't fit into those cubbyholes. Nurses need to write out their observations."

A: "You can fill the cubbyholes without looking at the patient."

RN: "That's exactly what happens. It's a check-off is all."

A: "The charts are standard and have nothing to do with a particular patient in a particular bed?"

RN: "Right. Not only is there only a flow sheet, but it's in the computer. When the doctor comes on the floor he has to deal with the computer, unless he can find the right nurse to inform him. How many doctors do you know have time to do that?"

A: "They could print it out and put it on the chart."

RN: "It's printed out after the patient is discharged."

A: "Why don't they print it out for the doctor?

RN: "Because they can't. The computer program is written so they can't print it out until the patient is discharged."

A: "Who made the decision that it would be done this way?"

RN: "Nursing administration, I guess."

Chapter Thirteen
ERRORS, TRAPS, AND ACCIDENTS

ERRORS AND ACCIDENTS

Hospital administrators, medical societies at all levels, insurance carriers, management experts, state and federal governments, and every concerned person and organization are looking for ways to limit the number of faults in the hospital and medical system.

The Joint Commission on Accreditation of Healthcare Organizations (JCAHO) inspects hospitals and other services related to medicine. It issues certificates of approval for those meeting set standards, and periodically sends out **Sentinel Events** alerts to stop harmful practices in the industry. In-depth information on this endeavor can be found by giving a search engine the simple title, "Sentinel Events." JCAHO defines SE as "… an unexpected occurrence involving death or serious physical or psychological injury, or the risk thereof."

Errors occur in small community hospitals, nursing homes, and doctors' offices, and regrettably in the more elite institutions as well. Tragic error made the headlines when Duke University surgeons transplanted live organs from a donor whose blood type did not match the recipient's, with fatal results. The State of New York fined Mount Sinai Hospital in Manhattan for the death of a partial liver donor. Government officials took action against Johns Hopkins University for the death of a volunteer in an asthma experiment. A surgeon at Memorial Sloan-Kettering Cancer Center operated on the wrong side of a patient's brain, and a 39-year-old woman died from an overdose of chemotherapy for breast cancer in a Harvard teaching institution. The information in this paragraph all came from published news.

Drug and food accidents are commonplace. An accident at the Binghamton nursery in 1959 made history. Salt was substituted for sugar in the infants' formula. The consequent high concentration of sodium in the bloodstream pulled an extreme amount of water out of the brain of each child. This caused the brain to shrink to a much smaller size, so constricted as to break bridging veins from the brain surface to the large drainage sinuses in the brain covering, adding the complication of bleeding and clot formation.

Faults are beyond the grasp of any one part of the system, or any single authority. Human error occurs at every level of mankind's endeavors. Only private vigilance and careful attention can prevent these deadly mistakes.

Self-protection is one of the driving forces of nature, and it normally works for everyone every moment of the day. Innate defense mechanisms temper any motion a person makes. The brain with its extensions throughout the body is responsible. Without this self-protection, a person would choke to death while swallowing food, fall down the stairs, drown in the bathtub, fall on the floor when lifting one foot to step into clothes, wreck the car before getting to the street, strangle in sleep, and crash into furniture and doorways. In fact, no one would survive any of the everyday activities taken for granted.

This self-protection operates beneath everyday awareness to guard life, and it is driven by the normal body chemistry. But drugs administered in the hospital or elsewhere can alter this chemistry. With some a person becomes less alert to danger, the innate defenses diminished or abolished, producing a passive and submissive state, even irresponsible silliness. Then the person belongs totally to the system unless someone is there to guard him.

There is another automatic form of protective behavior in everyday contact with people. Ordinarily no one rolls over for anybody. Clerks, cashiers, waiters, lawyers, and family members don't depersonalize anyone to a more manageable and submissive state of mind. Such arrogance would not be tolerated, and there is no defensible reason for it when a patient enters a hospital or a doctor's office, especially in the era of modern medicine. The entire system has become an immense and complicated industry growing out of control, and no doctor can know every facet of medicine. Each patient is just one more of his many, too often, too many. The availability of information in the twenty-first century empowers people to protect themselves in the medical system. But this precaution requires effort.

Medical mistakes are worse than other mistakes because the rules and restraints common to the rest of humanity do not govern medicine where privileges are beyond the ordinary. Despite the numerous checks and balances instituted in the system to control medicine as a practice and a profession, errors do occur. The vast majority of such errors are not a doctor's fault directly. They are faults of the system and how things are done.

In reality, does the doctor actually practice medicine? When did he ever draw a blood sample himself, give a patient a drug injection or vaccination, or bring his pills and tuck his patient in for the night? Probably never. Unless he performs surgery, the doctor does not practice medicine directly. He practices through pharmacists, nurses, nurses' aides, physiotherapists, and others, including the orderlies. In this hierarchy of direct one-on-one contact, the levels of authority, education, and skill diminish progressively, and the chances for errors increase. In this jungle a person becomes an entity unto himself, and no other person or system can bear full responsibility for his safety. Every person should have a right to self-preservation, even when surrendering certain privileges and privacy in order to receive medical treatment.

The medical industry has become increasingly complex and will become more so as it continues to evolve. Of course, no one has to be reminded of its miracles; millions of people who would have died at an early age in other times are alive today because of technological advances and the discovery of cures for particular diseases. Many of these people have come to depend on the new technology.

Frantic and hurried treatment is too often the necessary expedient. The bigger the crowd and the more hurried the activity, the greater are the chances for error. The genuinely ill may be passed over for needed treatment, and emergencies might get lost in the confusion of routine. Because of all the separate activities involved in treatment and management, the system serves anyone from its many parts, an arm at a time like the tentacles of an octopus, one coming from this direction, the next from another, and the patient might become of secondary importance to the routine. We've already said this, but we can't say it too many times: If all blame for faults of the hospital system could be placed on a single cause, it would be this reality—**no one is in charge**. Responsibility slips out of every hand involved.

The person too sick to take care of himself needs a family member at his bedside to protect against mishaps. Neither the able nor the weak should ever go into any jungle alone, whether it is a rainforest populated by predators and poisonous snakes or the man-made jungle, the modern medical complex. The analogy is apt enough to be taken soberly. There are many ways to kill a person in a hospital. In this medical jungle, anyone should have the right to self-preservation, and a defense against life-threatening confrontations. A life-saving medicine can become a fatal poison when misused. A life-saving operation can turn into an execution when done on the wrong person, on the wrong side of the right person, or by inept hands.

Failures occur in hospitals because of the air of infallibility and righteousness. Hospital personnel might think it won't or can't happen here. So what can they do to the unguarded? They can kill with the wrong medicine or wrong dosage, with neglect, and with the wrong diagnosis. They can scald in the bathtub, let a person fall out of a bed, and overdose with X-rays. They can operate on the wrong patient, do the wrong operation, remove the wrong arm or leg, and let someone bleed to death after surgery. They can cause a fatal infection, accidentally or carelessly inject air into arteries or veins, electrocute, strangle with restraints, and crush with an inflatable mattress. They can maim or kill in various other ways. They can be dead wrong, and a patient may be dead because they are wrong. Contrary to what people would like to think, these are not the hands of angels. They are hands of mere mortals, with the same fallibilities. As in any other place from bed to battlefield, the person is on his own. The remedy for this danger lies in precaution. Who will protect a patient who has to enter the system? A person's awareness of the need for self-preservation in the medical arena should be as keen as when he drives his car into traffic on a busy interstate highway. If he is too sick to know the difference, a family member or a friend should be there to think for him.

Every intern knows to check labels in all situations, but especially to check labels when giving a blood transfusion. A mistake here can be fatal. Regardless of how well the system works or despite a blood bank with a perfect record so far, the doctor never starts the blood running into a vein until he has double-checked identifying markers of the donor type, the patient type, the names, and all possibilities. An error would be the fault of the system, but the final responsibility falls on the person actually administering the transfusion.

So it should be with organ transplantation. For live organs, like heart and lung transplants, the donor and the recipient must have the same blood type. The surgeon who does not double-check the match himself is taking a risk. He complacently trusts the hospital system, and system failures will occur eventually. A wise and wily surgeon would never take such a chance, but one of the smartest and one of the best did. "Mistake" is the most it can be called, and the smartest, most committed people make them, too. Mistakes ruin lives, take lives, and lose ball games. Mistakes are always stupid. Mistakes occur where thinking stops.

In this particular instance, the patient got a second transplant and died anyway. Think of the cost. Both donors were wasted. Three hearts died, and two sick recipients were denied hearts, and they, too, died waiting. The heart team at the time of the first operation played another potentially lethal game of brinksmanship. While one team was in an airplane returning with the organs they had retrieved in another town, a second heart team had already taken the ailing heart out of the patient in order to have her ready for the transplant when the first team returned. What if the plane had crashed or had to be diverted because of weather? The recipient would have lost her last chance and died needlessly, and the donor heart would have met a futile death.

What can a member of a family do when caught up in either side of this tragic theater? First, don't yield to the heart team's high and mighty, and they are the highest and the mightiest. The lack of checking identity and the risk-taking with the airplane are invitations to tragedy, and betray their vulnerability. Under such circumstances, don't let anyone do such things. Find out about the donor, and don't allow an operation to be started until the donor organ is in the operating suite.

Tales of hospital accidents come from the doctors themselves. This one was from a dedicated and competent neurosurgeon, and he told it with great concern.

The patient, an 18-month-old hydrocephalic (water head) child from out in the country had not received proper treatment, and the head had become far too large. Trapped fluid in blocked pathways and ventricles (cavities of the brain) ballooned with too much fluid, stretching the brain to alarming thinness. The neurosurgeon decided to drain out some of the accumulating fluid to bring the head size down and relieve the severe brain-ballooning, this in preparation for a more permanent type of operation to shunt excess fluid to another part of the body.

He placed one end of a tube in a cavity of the brain (ventricle), and brought the other end out to a bag placed on a bedside table at the patient's body level. The arrangement relieved the excess pressure, but not too fast or too far. The operation went easily enough, and everybody turned to the business of the day. Later, someone entered the room and found the drainage bag on the floor and the child dead.

How did the bag get on the floor? It was not the child's fault. Its head was too big for free movement and its hands had been restrained. All the fluid from the brain ran into the bag once it was lowered below the brain level, and the brain collapsed. Bedside vigilance would have prevented the incident.

This is the account of another mistake as told by an emergency room nurse. In the late evening hours the ER had quieted to a lull after frantic activity over the victims of an automobile accident. A well-dressed, middle-aged woman entered the area and hurriedly approached the receptionist, who was busy on the telephone, the receiver cradled between a raised shoulder and a cheek. The receptionist ignored the intruder and continued her conversation, eyes downcast. The middle-aged woman looked like a business executive, neatly dressed in a double-breasted suit, and from her manner seemed to be accustomed to giving orders and tolerating no slack. She hesitated, but not more than a second as she realized the telephone conversation was personal and unrelated to any kind of emergency room business. Then she interrupted and demanded to know the whereabouts of her husband. The receptionist said, "Just a minute," into the phone, placed it on the desktop, and haughtily proceeded to scan a clipboard, running her ballpoint down a column of entries. Without looking up she said, "Mr. Fry was placed in cubicle ten. You have to take a seat in the lounge and wait for the doctor."

"How long has Mr. Fry been here?" asked Mrs. Fry.

The receptionist, already picking up the phone, heaved an impatient sigh, ran the ballpoint down another column on the pad, and said, "Two hours ago, 10:30." She looked up and officiously pointed in a direction behind Mrs. Fry. "The waiting room is over there."

Mrs. Fry eyed the double row of cubicles behind the receptionist's desk. The room had grown too quiet. Mrs. Fry walked around the desk and down the row of cubicles, until she parted the drapes on number ten. She came out immediately, and all hell broke loose. Mrs. Fry had found Mr. Fry quite dead, entirely alone in cubicle ten, fully dressed in his street clothes with his shoes on.

The following story, pieced together later, is both ridiculous and sad. Mr. Fry walked into the emergency room with his left hand clasped to his chest. He presented his complaint, a tight feeling over his heart, a burning in his gullet, pain radiating down his left arm, beginning all of a sudden while on his way to the airport for another important business flight. His symptoms had been getting worse steadily, and he swung by the ER in a state of fear. The receptionist made him take a seat and fill out a form. After some delay she directed him to cubicle 10 and turned to notify a doctor just as the outside door burst open, and a gurney bearing a bloody form rolled in, pushed by a shuffling and hurrying ambulance crew. Another followed, and a helicopter landed with more. The frantic activity lasted for another hour. Then all grew quiet, and the doctor had nothing to do. In fact, he returned in a state of boredom to a well-worn copy of an old *Life* magazine. No one had told him about the patient in cubicle ten, who had not been seen since he disappeared behind the drapes unescorted.

The ER staff forgot Mr. Fry, and he died alone at the very place he should have been getting help. Could such a thing happen in a modern emergency room? It did, and Mr. Fry probably could have been saved. Clot-dissolving drugs administered soon after the onset of a heart attack could have saved his life. Emergency stents are saving even more victims. Mr. Fry did the wise thing by coming to the emergency room as soon as his symptoms became convincing, but the hospital system failed him. He had been traveling alone with no one along for protection.

Some of the routine and commonplace techniques in the medical scene carry dangers, among them the subclavian line in particular. Invasion of the human body is not to be taken lightly, not even a tiny skin nick. When deeper structures must be entered blindly, the dangers arise accordingly. Getting a catheter correctly placed in an invisible and non palpable vein is not easy.

The vein can be felt with neither needle nor finger tip, and the beginner will tend to probe around a bit. The needle may accidentally go into the subclavian artery, which lies right behind the vein. This is not where it should be. Another complication, a punctured lung causing air to escape into the chest cavity (pneumothorax) is commonplace, although usually no serious consequences occur in the long run.

As an example of some of the dangers, here is an all too real incident. One morning, the assignment for a subclavian line went to a doctor in training, a brilliant fellow but one known for an inability to use his hands skillfully. He inserted the subclavian line on the patient's right side and hooked up an IV of clear fluid, set it dripping, and went about his business. The patient, a 36 year-old woman, had been sick for a long time with complications of a ruptured appendix. The subsequent peritonitis led to several abscesses, one behind the liver, required multiple operations. At last, after many months, she seemed to be healing, but she had shrunk to skin and bones. The senior medical resident decided to give her hyper-alimentation (a thick combination of various proteins, sugars, other nutrients and vitamins) feedings into her veins, and hoped to send her home soon. Her five young children needed her.

The medication nurse came along sometime after the subclavian line had been inserted, with a 50cc syringe full of this stuff for the first feeding. She shut off the drip, inserted the syringe tip into the hub of the subclavian line, and rapidly injected the entire contents of the syringe. Almost instantly the patient gasped and went limp, and her breathing stopped.

Post-mortem examination (autopsy) found the catheter in the artery, not the vein. It had been threaded down into the main artery above the heart (the aorta) where the heart empties the blood flowing toward the head and out to the body. All the blood vessels to the brain get their blood supply through arterial branches in the upper wall of this great vessel. The violent stream of blood swept the tip of the catheter up the left carotid artery, and the entire bolus of thick viscid fluid had been injected directly into the brain blood supply. The patient died of a massive stroke. The fluid should have been placed in the great veins going to the heart, where it would have been mixed and diluted before going to the arteries and out to smaller vessels.

One dangerous break in technique followed another to compound this tragedy. The person who placed the catheter should have recognized the difference between arterial and venous blood. The person who injected the fluid should have pulled blood back on the syringe plunger first, and the sight of bright red blood would have been warning enough. Injection of anything should be done in slow increments, and the patient closely observed for adverse reactions.

The subclavian device carries other dangers, as in an accident with another patient, John Olden(not his real name). His son arrived at the hospital at 7 a.m. to take his father home. The doctor had been optimistic about Olden's recovery and promised to discharge him at 7:30. As the son entered the room, Mr. Olden sat up in bed to speak, but instead he gasped and fell over to one side. The son ran for help, and by the time the nurses got to the room, Olden was dead.

John Olden had been healthy until a week before when his horse kicked him in the shin, breaking both bones below the knee. The horse manure in the torn flesh over the bone fragments frightened the doctor into administering massive doses of antibiotics to prevent gas gangrene, flesh-eating bacteria, and other infections. This required a subclavian line, according to medical opinion. Mr. Olden, a tough 75-year-old, had never taken a painkiller, sleeping pills, or a sedative of any kind in his life. The drugs hit him hard and caused a state of restless euphoria. He was out of it most of the time, and not unhappy. On his last night in the hospital, he somehow worked the line loose at the hub of the needle in the catheter near its entry point through the skin. When he sat up, the line fell out, leaving the catheter in the vein wide open.

How could this kill him? The answer lies in the veins deep in the body. These vessels return blood to the heart at a very low pressure, compared to the pressure in the arteries. The pressure varies from about zero to numbers down in the minus range, depending on the gravitational position of a particular vein. When a person lies down, the pressure in the veins inside the chest registers about zero, but when he sits up it plunges. In the case of Olden, the negative pressure sucked a large volume of air through the open catheter into the veins, and Mr. Olden died of massive air embolism. Was this a preventable death? Of course it was. A massive air embolus can be fatal without crossing over into the arterial blood by one of several mechanisms, like blocking the flow of blood from the heart to the lungs, and by damage to the lungs.

Besides the described dangers of subclavian (central venous) lines: the fatal bleeding from the outer end of the catheter, the fatal air embolism, the fatal injection into the wrong vessel, and air in the chest from faulty puncturing efforts, other accidents happen. These include bleeding into the chest cavity from faulty needle placement, punctured nerves supplying the arm, and damage to major arteries in the neck: the carotid and the subclavian (under the collarbone). Punctured heart wall from threading the catheter too far down causes violent bleeding between the outer heart wall and its covering sac, the pericardium, and this bleeding rapidly compresses the heart fatally (cardiac tamponade) unless discovered and treated. The catheter may be pushed through the heart valve into the big vessel carrying blood from the heart to the lung (pulmonary artery) causing rupture of the artery, or leading to the injection of fluids and drugs into the wrong place.

The catheter may be pushed through the wall of the vein and empty the fluids it carries into tissues of the neck or chest. The catheter can itself be lost down the lumen of the vessel, so can the wire used to help guide the catheter in at the time of its insertion. These constitute two additional kinds of embolism. Damage can be done to a major lymphatic vessel (the third circulation system, arteries and veins being the other two), resulting in a collection of lymphatic fluid in the neck or chest, a leak most difficult to stop.

Then there is the complication of infection, as already described. An indwelling catheter or needle opens the body to all the risks of the outside environment. The most careful technique should be used to guard against bacterial contamination. Infections will occur, and these can vary from skin inflammation to a fatal septicemia.

Certain very practical precautions should be taken. The correct use of X-ray pictures or the use of the fluoroscope will ensure accurate placement of the catheter tip. If the catheter after its placement produces a slow flow of dark blood, it is in a venous supply of blood; rapid flow of bright red blood indicates arterial positioning. YouTube shows all the details.

Concern over the incidence of complications of central venous lines has prompted the FDA and various manufacturers of medical equipment to release educational videotapes entitled *Central Venous Catheter Complications*, available from the National Audiovisual Center, 8700 Edgeworth Drive, Capitol Heights, MD 20743-3701; telephone (800) 788-6282.

The patient or the bedside guardian can protect against the hazards of a central venous line (subclavian line). Talk to the attending surgeon about who is to place the line, and object to a greenhorn doing this procedure without proper supervision at the bedside, probing for a vein he is having a hard time finding. After this otherwise minor surgical procedure and assuming the line has been placed by competent hands and double-checked for accuracy, someone still should watch for complications. Any change in the patient's condition, including swelling in the neck, hoarseness, shortness of breath, fever, rapid pulse, pallor, sweating, loss of consciousness, calls for intervention. Stop the flow of fluid and get help.

Operating room accidents are beyond the reach of both the patient and guardians. Some of the after effects can lead to the discovery of an unrecognized complication; lost operating room equipment in surgical wounds happens 1,500 times a year in United States hospitals, according to one count (Gawande, Atul A., see multiple references on the Internet), and in fact, probably more often, many never recognized and some not reported. Equipment left in wounds can be anything from fingernail size sponges to four-inch squares of gauze and cloths the size of kitchen towels, and surgical instruments of any size. Continued unexplained pain or failure to improve warrants investigation to rule out this possibility. A plain X-ray picture of the wound area, usually the abdominal cavity, is the first step. Instruments will be obvious; some but not all fabrics used in an operation have X-ray markers for identification. Retained foreign objects stimulate extensive scarring and lead to infection. Corrosion of metal instruments in body tissue may cause inflammation and ultimate rejection. The possibility of something having been left in the wound should be investigated when the patient fails to thrive.

Errors in preoperative management lead to surgical tragedies. Vomiting in the operating room at the time of induction of the anesthetic or during the operation can cause serious and often fatal complications, such as suffocation on aspirated material or chemical pneumonia from digestive fluids. Usually this happens when the patient has been given breakfast by mistake. Some patients assume it's okay to eat the food since it has been brought to the bedside, an error made by the people designated to carry trays, or by the person responsible for the written orders. The answer, "Bacon and eggs," too often surprises the anesthesiologist who has learned to ask his 7:30 a.m. patient what he had for breakfast. The answer should be "nothing." The order is or should be written NPO, nothing peros, or nothing by mouth after a certain time, usually midnight. The stomach should be empty of food when a patient goes to the operating room.

TRAPS
SIDE RAILS RESTRAINTS, CASTS, DRESSINGS, HIGH BEDS, HOSPITAL MURDER

Side rails, as previously stated, are hazards, while at best they keep the rational patient from accidentally falling out of bed. Raised rails beside an obstreperous patient in restraints create a deathtrap. A confused patient hell-bent on escape will go over the top of the rails, thus increasing the distance of a fall to the floor. Going through a rail can be worse. Accidents are commonplace, and they happen something like this: Old Jake Gregory finally stopped cursing and yelling about 3 o'clock in the morning. The young nurse on the ward felt relieved to be rid of the noise. Thank goodness his medicine had taken effect, and he had gone to sleep. The silence seemed almost creepy, but she went about her business and forgot him. At 6:30 morning rounds, Gregory's bed looked odd from a distance, and when the nurses approached, he seemed to be hugging the rail, wrapped in the covers. A nurse pulled down the sheet and jumped back with a little squeal. Not a pretty sight there in the railings, Gregory's neck twisted, his body nearly out of bed between bottom rung and mattress, chest hanging over the side, his chin caught on a rung, suspending his body toward the floor, his hands still in restraints, his limbs stiff as a board. His blue-blotched face told the story. He was dead, garroted in the rails.

Jake Gregory was a house painter. They drink a lot, so people say. His fall 20 feet from a ladder at work broke several ribs and face bones, caused multiple cuts and bruises, and the impact knocked him unconscious for a few hours. He was getting well from his injuries but became confused and began demanding whiskey. He did not have DTs but he was accustomed to his drink every day. He didn't get whiskey, and the symptoms of dependency began to show. No one paid attention, and he was transferred out of SCU because he was making too much noise. The nurse there was in collusion with the night supervisor, and so she easily got permission to be rid of the nuisance. This preventable death would not have happened in the SCU where his bed stood in full view of the nurses' station. It would not have happened if the resident on the clinic service had been wise enough to give Gregory a shot of whiskey with his evening meal, or if a guardian had been by his bedside.

Mistakes in the everyday management of flesh wounds cause complications of varying degrees. Dressings, bandages, casts, and braces can create problems when too tight or otherwise incorrectly applied. Pain developing in the hidden area under a dressing or a cast calls for investigation. Change of skin color, too white or too blue, or increased swelling in a limb means the dressing is too tight and is interfering with blood circulation. Check the areas beyond the dressing, like the toes and fingers, for color changes. Don't wait until the next day. Blue toes or fingers, blanching toes or fingers mean danger. Waiting until morning to release the cast or dressing can cause loss of the limb. Here is an example: The patient, a middle-aged woman, was screaming with severe pain beneath her dressing on the night following an operation on the right side of her head. She was fully alert, with no damage to the brain. A careful house officer removed the dressing. It had been wound around and around her head, creating a neat white turban. And a good thing he did remove it. The person who applied the dressing had bent the right ear forward and bound it down tightly. The ear had turned deep blue with hints of impeding blackness. As the dressing came off, the ear began to turn pink. If the ear had spent the night captured in the faulty dressing, it would have been dead by morning.

Here is another common trap, the patient's bed. Why is it up in the air, at least three feet from the floor? Certainly not for the patient; it's an old custom for the convenience of the hospital staff. They don't have to stoop so far to reach the patient for medications, food trays, changing linens, and the patient's clothes. Then, the space underneath served in the old days for placing chamber pots, urinals, and the like. Add the side rail when elevated and secured in place, and the patient can increase the distance of his fall to the floor by another 18 inches. Confused and agitated patients will crawl out of bed and fall. And these falls are often fatal. Restraints appear on the scene, bringing another deadly hazard.

Such a patient needs a doctor who will get to the cause of the agitation, usually related to discomfort or pain. If the cause can be found and treated, the problem of dangerous behavior will go away or diminish significantly. If not, then sedation and restraints become the order of the day. Therein lie many hazards. Restraints may make the confused and resistant patient more manageable, but such devices also create several dangers, including interference with breathing. Flat on his back, the patient may strangle on fluids and junk collecting in his throat, and with his hands tied he can only spit into the open, provided he is conscious enough to try to stay alive. He may suffocate flat on his belly. Supine, he can worm too far down under the edge of a body restraint, engage the throat, and obstruct his airway. Increasing the sedation if the patient becomes more unmanageable may endanger the patient's life. Towels or cloths placed over the patient's head when he is biting and spitting can cause suffocation. In fact, there are dozens of variations on this dismal and frustrating theme. The one thing this patient needs most is constant attendance by people who care about him.

Preventative measures include using low beds, withholding orders not to restrain until absolutely necessary, treating the symptoms, talking to the patient, and never restraining or sedating to punish agitated behavior. The patient will not remember this terrible episode in his life when he recovers. His behavior is beyond his voluntary control, and he is totally at the mercy of those around him.

Fire is an added hazard to smokers. They will light up if they get their hands on matches or lighters, and a confused, desperate patient may try to burn the restraints.

Older people especially, and others in a weak or confused state from illness and medication, are in danger of falling when they get out of bed for a trip to the bathroom. Pride and disobedience compound the problem in older patients. But falls can also occur down the stairs, out of windows, down laundry chutes, or the patient might wander off and fall from a balcony or roof.

Murder in the Hospital

This is indeed another trap. Hospital murderers have been convicted the world over. Authorities have detected doctors, nurses, hospital employees, wandering strangers, and members of patients' families among the guilty. A hospital, especially a big charity institution, understaffed during the late hours of the night, offers an opportunity for murder like no other place. Not even a dark alley with no one else around affords the murderer such a chance. A terminally ill patient, a sick patient, or an old patient found dead in bed is no big surprise and raises few questions or suspicions. On the Contrary, finding a person dead in the street would stop traffic, attract a crowd, summon the police, bring in an ambulance with a rescue squad, and a need to know what happened.

The killer may use a pillow to suffocate, especially those too weak and sick to offer resistance. But the most frequent method involves drugs. The patient unguarded in a room or a cubicle alone with an IV drip running is a perfect target. The smart killer might employ a larger dose of the same drug the patient is already getting, like one of the digitalis derivatives used to treat heart failure and abnormal heart rhythms. Many heart patients are chronically overdosed anyway, and a little more pushes them over the brink, sudden, quiet death not a surprise.

Another poorly regulated drug, insulin, becomes lethal in large doses. Potassium chloride in the right amount will almost instantly stop the heart, yet it is a part of all life-supporting solutions being fed into a vein. A few drops of curare or one of its relatives or modern descendents (like Pavulon), used in anesthesia to paralyze muscle action, stops respiration, and the patient smothers to death. The transfusion of mismatched blood, the infusion of the wrong fluid, a too rapid infusion of the otherwise right fluid, or too much of any one of numerous drugs can be fatal.

People intent on killing use these or other drugs including adrenaline, heroin, morphine, and barbiturates. Medical serial killers are caught now and then, but their numbers as revealed in reference sources are alarming.

No doubt many hospital and nursing home killings are never discovered. Total prevention of fatal drug accidents and hospital murders is not possible, but bedside vigilance will do much to stop the abuses.

The remedy here once again is vigilance, constant attendance the best prevention. It can spare or diminish the need for restraints. All hospital injuries are preventable. Mental aberrations secondary to suffering may be aggravated by sedation and mind-altering drugs; treatment of the underlying cause of the symptoms will restore a more normal pattern of behavior. Old people in nursing homes too often do not receive adequate medical treatment. For instance, recurrent urinary bladder infections torment old women especially. The misery of burning, stinging urgency and almost constant voiding of urine drives them crazy, and the result may be dangerous agitation and noisy behavior. Treatment with the proper medication brings quick relief. But what happens? The nurse gets on the telephone after she has had enough of the difficulty with old Mrs. Becker on a Sunday afternoon shift and tells the doctor, "Mrs. Becker is noisy and screaming and confused, and we can't do a thing with her." She says nothing about the patient's other symptoms, nor does she remind the doctor of Mrs. Becker's frequent bouts of urinary bladder infection. The doctor is not about to look in on the old woman himself. He orders a sedative, like Haldol. This drug in particular causes an unusual reaction in Mrs. Becker. She gets crazier, in fact psychotic, and has no idea what she is doing or tying to do. Louder screaming, greater agitation, falling out of bed, getting out of bed and falling, collapsing in the bathroom in a puddle of discharged fecal matter, are among the manifestations. The personnel then get an order to restrain her, where she becomes a total helpless prisoner to her suffering unless some sensible person comes to her rescue. A member of the family would know her bladder infection history and insist on the proper treatment.

And how does a family member get the attention needed when interference becomes necessary? Expect resistance and an attitude. Start with the nurse's aide, or the nurse in charge, but don't waste too much time at either level. Somewhere in the building there is a head nurse's office. Go there, next or first depending on your previous difficulties with the same sort of problem. Keep going if you have too. Call the doctor retained by the home to treat ill patients. Call the hospital administrator if you need to, even if he is at home on a weekend. As a last resort, call your lawyer.

Chapter Fourteen
THE EMERGENCY ROOM

Any patient who appears in the emergency room with a real emergency must be accommodated. This is the law. But, people do take advantage of emergency rooms for various reasons. Some do not have and cannot afford a primary care physician, or don't know how to go about finding help in the medical world. Working parents may have no time for access to treatment until after their working hours, and this excuse is abused by people who simply don't want to take responsibility of health maintenance. Any emergency room in a big city hospital is always mobbed with the really sick and the grievously injured, but also with bums and deadbeats, addicts looking for drugs, the homeless looking for shelter, and the suddenly ill who don't know where else to turn. It is a last resort for the penniless, the uninsured, the unemployed, and the desperate.

No democracy exerts itself in the emergency room, because death is entirely autocratic. If a patient is not dying or obviously is in no immediate danger of dying he will have to wait, maybe hours before getting attention. Between lulls, the ER is a scene of blood and gore, with frantic and too often frenzied activity. There is no time for comprehensive evaluation of non-emergency health problems.

Emergency rooms should be for emergencies only. Abusing them by congesting the waiting room with the indigent and other social problems only dilutes their real quality and hampers the purpose. Emergency medicine is now a specialty, and most big emergency rooms are manned around the clock by these specially trained physicians. Staff specialists are on call for emergencies in their fields. But the emergency room is the last place to go if it can be avoided. Only when circumstances force the issue should anyone appear in an emergency room unknown and without referral. Under these circumstances the patient is entirely at the mercy of the system and has to take what he gets. The primary care physician may choose to meet in the ER with one of his patients stricken at home after hours.

Rescue squads responding to 911 calls by law must go to the nearest emergency room, and the nearest ER to any one patient may be inferior to one further away. Once a person is on this route the die is cast. Although emergency room personnel are not allowed to refuse treatment to a true emergency, the doctors may refer a patient to another center better equipped to handle certain problems, like trauma. The flat refusal to treat an indigent patient with an emergency problem is a federal offense, and this applies to the specialist who refuses to come to the emergency room when he is called.

The remedy here is to avoid emergency rooms if at all possible: The person who faces a serious problem in a strange city, in an emergency room, lost and frightened for himself or a family member, would do well to call his physician back home. More than likely he will know someone whose staff can come to the stranded person's aid.

If the personnel appear to have forgotten, are being too slack, or do not recognized the seriousness of the problem, go to the receptionist and begin inquiries. If a friend or relative has been behind the curtains too long, with no word coming back, the guardian should start asking questions.

Many hospitals and medical centers have a list of patient's rights, including emergency room treatment, available in printed form or posted on the Web. Use an Internet search engine like Google to find the information for the hospital nearest you.

Chapter Fifteen
THE BRAIN DEAD AND EUTHANASIA

This special niche in medicine is fraught with both error and mischief, as in this instance in the early days of the transplant era, where the doctor on duty in the emergency room worked himself into a state of high excitement over what he took to be a brain death. In the circumstances, he was guilty of enthusiasm, one of the worst and most dangerous traits a doctor can develop. Enthusiasm and judgment run counter to each other.

He thought he had a brain-dead patient on his hands, and he could see his name in the newspapers for sending a donor to New York by helicopter. He also thought of himself as the modern man, intelligent and immensely practical. New York desperately needed a heart for a celebrity of the same blood type. But the doctor had to have a second opinion, a safeguard set up by wiser people.

The second opinion came from a neurosurgeon on call for the night. He went to the hospital, entered the emergency room, and walked up to the so-called brain-dead patient, Tim Jones. The neurosurgeon's reaction was immediate and hot. He started commanding and took over the emergency room. Nurses and interns rushed to help. Tim Jones had been shot in the head with a .20 gauge shotgun at too close a range for the shot to have scattered, and the round bolus acting as a single missile took out a piece of skull, the muscle in the temple, and a piece of the temporal lobe of the brain. The patient was unconscious, gasped occasionally, and had no blood pressure. The neurosurgeon went to work, delivering more orders. Fluids were poured into the veins, and a transfusion started. The ER doctor interfered. "Doctor," he said to the surgeon, "The patient is brain dead, and we are wasting precious time. A helicopter is waiting for the harvested organs. I didn't call you down here to treat the dead, I called for you to supply the required second opinion."

The surgeon quelled an impulse to retaliate, and replied, "Get the hell out of my way!" He rushed the patient to the operating room, stopped the bleeding, patched the hole in the brain cover and skull, and closed the scalp with a sliding graft.

Six weeks later the patient, already back to work as a carpenter, paid his third visit to the neurosurgeon's office. The surgeon said, "You are in the clear now. You will never chew as well as you once could because the shotgun took away one of your major chewing muscles. When you're driving and have to make a left turn, cut your head sharply to the left. You have lost half the vision in each eye, the temple side on the left and the nose side on the right from damage to a part of the temporal lobe of your right brain.

Other than those problems, you are very much will be for some time."

Except for the checks and balances written in regulations for establishing the diagnoses of brain death, and the wisdom of a second opinion, poor Tim's heart would be beating in another man's body. After all, he **had** been shot in the head; he was unconscious and bleeding terribly, and the family had already assumed the worst. They would have accepted whatever the medical personnel in the emergency room told them. The emergency room doctor did not get to be a hero. His dreams of glory were shattered. But, he was not practicing the tenets of good medicine taught by his mentors. You could not call him intellectually dishonest, just intellectually disobedient. And he made a terrible and fundamental misdiagnosis: The patient was not unconscious from brain damage; he was unconscious from shock due to blood loss.

The term brain death legalizes the procurement of living organs for transplantation, particularly the heart, lungs, liver, and digestive tract. Brain death, however, does not amount to real death. The brain is not actually dead, yet. True, a large part of it is gone forever, but some of it still functions, otherwise the heart would stop. But the part responsible for breathing and any kind of recognizable awareness, the perception of pain, and response to stimuli from the outside world has stopped working forever.

Certain people call this patient legally dead, but the patient certainly is not dead, not yet. However, the patient may be dead legally shortly thereafter through a natural course of events or from the process of taking live organs, or from simply cutting off the machine supporting breathing. A more aggressive doctor who does not want to be bothered with niceties declares the patient dead while the heart still beats. This doctor will sometimes tell the family the patient is dead, and then the transplant team proceeds with removal of live organs. A doctor like this considers himself immensely practical and does not want a distinction between death and brain death, and claims there is no difference. But the distinction nevertheless exists. Leave nature to itself, and putrefaction immediately begins after death, but not in the state of brain death. Said in another way, the dead rot, the brain-dead do not. Brain death is a contrivance of mankind; death itself most certainly is not.

The diagnosis of brain death relies entirely on clinical findings. No test, laboratory or otherwise, can prove the diagnosis. Certain findings always must be present. First, the patient is unconscious or comatose, as the doctors and nurses call it. Second, the patient is dependent on a respirator, mechanical breathing, for his breath of life. If this support stops, the heart will also stop within a few minutes. Third, as a part of the unconscious condition, the patient shows no response to any stimulus, painful or otherwise. Fourth, the pupils of the eyes are fully wide open and fixed, and do not close even to the strongest direct light.

If all of these conditions are present, is the patient brain dead? Not necessarily. Other conditions, not always fatal, can and do cause these findings. Shock from blood loss as death draws near, as in the case of Tim Jones' narrow escape, deceptively mimics brain death. Profound lowering of body temperature (hypothermia) from exposure to cold can imitate brain death almost to perfection. Dehydration along with abnormalities of the sodium, potassium, and sugar levels in the bloodstream can produce a state resembling death. Deep sedation from any number of drugs can produce all the findings at the end stages just before real death.

In the history of mankind's struggle with the determination of the time of death, there are hair-raising tales of people being accidentally buried alive. They were not dead, despite the doctor's declaration otherwise. They awoke in the black grave in a state of panic, and then really did die from suffocation. Someone contrived the idea of burying the so-called dead with a cord stretching to a bell outside the grave. If the buried person came to life, he rang the bell, and a quick exhumation saved him, thus the phrase, "saved by the bell."

Certain tests support the clinical diagnosis of brain death. If pictures (arteriograms) of the main blood supply to the brain show no blood flowing through the brain hemispheres, then the condition called brain death undoubtedly exists if all the other criteria are present, but the study is not specific. A brain wave tracing (EEG) showing no activity—a flat tracing—supports the diagnosis, but only because it does not refute it. The diagnosis cannot rest on this finding alone because the same tracing can be due to a fault in the system, like a dead wall socket, a malfunctioning machine, or an incorrect hook-up. On the Contrary, an active tracing can be made from a mold of gelatin in the highly charged electric atmosphere of a busy ICU. The diagnosis of brain death always rests ultimately on the clinical findings.

There should no great hurry to declare a patient brain dead. Life at this level can be maintained by support measures long enough for deliberate and considered action. Certain exceptions can and do occur. For instance, the person with the top of the head and brain torn off in a traffic accident, with all the clinical criteria of brain death, can be declared brain dead and become an immediate donor with no doubt about the wisdom of the decision. Patients with gunshot wounds of the brain producing immediate coma and respirator dependence likewise have suffered irreversible injury and will never benefit from treatment. Otherwise, in the absence of such doubtless evidence, both the doctor and the family should take time to be deliberate in the decision, and make the final call only after the diagnosis has been established beyond a reasonable doubt.

The specter of the hovering vulture accompanies the officious clerk-type who appears during emergency room efforts to save the grievously injured, with the question, "Doctor, are you going to declare this patient?" This question has changed the entire tone of emergency treatment of people who appear to be fatally injured but are not yet dead. Some of these patients can be saved with quick and appropriate treatment. The paramedic or nurse employed by an organ procurement outfit should not be allowed on the scene until the doctor in charge has exhausted all possibilities and has had a chance to talk to the patient's family.

None of these cautions are meant to interfere with the giving of live organs by the families of the truly brain dead. There could be no greater gift than the gift of extended life to another person who would otherwise die, and it gives continued life to a part of the condemned donor. It lets his heart live on. Just be careful and thorough.

To avoid trouble here, in the unfortunate and grievous position of having to make this decision for a relative, don't be hurried by anyone. Insist on treatment first (with the noted exception), and don't accept the brain death declaration without the proper evaluation by a qualified specialist, such as a neurosurgeon or neurologist. Don't let emergency medical people make this decision without the ultimate consultation. Brain death, as the term is used to justify the taking of live organs, usually comes from brain damage due to physical injury (automobiles, motorcycles, and gunshots), or from a fatal spontaneous brain hemorrhage. Be sure the state of the patient is not due to a drug overdose, alcohol and exposure to cold, loss of blood (shock), electrolyte and blood gas abnormalities, starvation, or a combination of treatable causes.

Euthanasia, Living Will, No Code

At the beginning of the transplant era, the responsibility for redefining death in order to support the new supply-line of organs was shirked to the doctors who rightfully refused the burden. The responsibility then became the moral duty of society as a whole, not the physician's alone, and over a period of years, state laws established guidelines. Unfortunately, the brain death concept has changed the tone of emergency room handling of head injury patients. It invites categorical conceptions, premature decisions, and consequent dreadful errors in treatment, a life cut short when it might have been saved.

The term "No Code" means not to resuscitate when the patient's heart fails, and this order is fraught with error. The idea is to prevent reflex and brutal attempts at cardiac resuscitation on a terminally ill patient who has finally died after all treatment has failed. In circumstances where the treatment plan is still developing and the prognosis uncertain, the question should not come up. When an officious type with pen and pad at ready interferes and approaches the doctor with the question, "Do you want a no code on this patient?" the doctor's outraged response is entirely justified. Code has saved many lives, and it should not be denied to a patient who has even the slightest chance of recovery. No one can accurately separate these from the hopeless until the patient fails to respond to all reasonable treatment.

Further into this morass, society has to deal with physician-assisted suicide and voluntary euthanasia. The suicide performs the act with the means supplied by a doctor. Voluntary euthanasia is a death-causing act performed by the doctor. Strong efforts are being made to legalize both, and certain doctors have acquired notoriety by defying existing law under the guise of mercy. What justifies these deaths? Ostensibly, pain and suffering lead the patient to prefer death. But according to several studies, pain is the primary factor in less than a third of the cases. More often the requests have been motivated by depression, hopelessness, mental distress, fear of being a burden and nuisance to the family, and a sense of solitude and abandonment. Most of the person's anguish comes from grief, the great suffering from worry, and from no one caring. Information in depth on this dilemma is available on Web sites, with special reference to the article, **Physician-Assisted Suicide: The Influence of Psychological Issues,** by William Breitbart, M.D., and Barry D. Rosenfeld, Ph.D. What a shame to put someone to death when a show of love, a word of care and reassurance, or other demonstrations of social support might well change the patient's attitude.

In our modern era, drugs are available to treat the pain and suffering of hopeless and terminal states. In the days before the psychoactive drugs (changing the psychological activity of the brain), physicians sometimes resorted to prefrontal lobotomy to relieve the suffering from widespread metastatic cancer, especially the intense pain from bone invasion. The operation changed the personality, but relieved the anguish of suffering and dying. Pain still persisted to a degree, but it did not make any difference to the patient. Drugs or a combination of drugs available now from a vast field of psychopharmacology (changing brain function with drug treatment) accomplish the same thing, and other drugs can be added to the regimen to relieve pain. Marijuana will alleviate the pain and suffering of cancer patients, as well as the nausea caused by chemotherapy, but has no proven effect on the cancer itself. Imagine society's accepting assisted suicide and refusing legalized marijuana to alleviate the symptoms of cancer.

The younger depressed patient with no terminal illness who wants to die or thinks he does, or says so without knowing what he really means, should be rescued. He needs psychiatric evaluation and treatment. The doctor who assists this patient with suicide in any way instead of offering a guiding hand out of the mental trap becomes guilty of the worst imaginable malpractice, the betrayal of his oath to patients and to medicine.

There may be a need in extreme and rare situations for voluntary euthanasia, but the involvement of doctors alone in the decision seems reprehensible. This somber act, disguised as suicide, should be a responsibility of society at large. A doctor has been trained to treat the sick, and the Hippocratic oath directs him to do no harm. His duty should be the ease of suffering, the treatment of both the patient and the disease. It is regrettable to see him become an executioner, and he should not let himself fall victim to this trap. Once he steps over these boundaries, would anyone want him as a personal physician?

The decision to kill a patient should be made by representatives of society at large, a committee of experts familiar with the problems. In the rare case of failure to obtain satisfactory relief with medications and humane care, the executioner should be anyone but a doctor of medicine. The doctor who tries to establish himself as a type of crusader in this macabre endeavor deserves the suspicion and distrust of his patients. Mercy can be brought to most of these people in a much kinder way. You might be able to rescue your own relative or friend with words of reassurance for the mental anguish, and with the right medication for relief of physical pain, and with your presence by his bedside.

LIVING WILL

The definition of a Living Will states, "a living will is a document which lets you decide whether or not to be kept on artificial life support" (see **www.legalzoom.com**). So worded, the document should not interfere with emergency treatment or confuse anyone about what to do. The will says, "not to be kept on." It says nothing about not using accepted emergency measures initially when an emergency arises. In most emergencies, the doctor cannot know the result of treatment until he has treated the patient. Once the situation stabilizes and the patient proves to be irretrievably dependent on life support measures, then is the time to honor the patient's living will and the family's wishes. Short cuts to this stage invite fatal mistakes.

Chapter Sixteen
THE SITUATION

On first view of the evidence, anyone would naturally wonder how the various concerned organizations came upon the numbers of preventable deaths in the system. Certainly they must have used some sort of approximation technique because such a head-by-head count would be virtually impossible in the vast medical and hospital system of this country. The Institute of Medicine of the National Academy of Science made estimates through a review of records in various states of the union. Adverse effects were found to have occurred in 2.9 percent (Colorado) to 3.7 (New York) percent. 6.6 percent to 13.6 percent of these events led to death, over half due to preventable medical errors. When these figures were extrapolated to the 33.6 million U.S. hospital admissions in one year (1997), the results varied state by state for a national total of somewhere between 44,000 and 97,000 preventable deaths yearly. Sources for drug (100,000) and the infection (100,000) deaths per year have already been cited. These figures, of course, have to be approximate, but the problem is, nevertheless, all too real.

Every person and organization concerned with medicine wants to improve this situation. Without doubt, enhancing and correcting the performance of people who work in the hospital system could eliminate some if not most accidents and mistakes, but it *is* a system, and a gargantuan one, without centralized leadership. Nor would the whole of medicine lend itself to such control. The king of the jungle certainly can't watch all the snakes.

Actually, the whole hospital system is about the doctor. Without the doctors, there would be no gigantic healthcare endeavor. All of this great industry exists because of the tremendous advances made during the past 60 years in the discovery of drugs and the development of technology. The doctor works in the system, but not for it. The doctor and the system thrive on each other, and no one is really the boss.

One doctor has privileges to practice in a particular hospital and so do other members of the medical staff. From the standpoint of quality control of individual performance no one with real power runs the open-staff hospital. Usually, each year members of a particular department, like urology or general surgery, elect a new chief, and he serves for only the one year. The authority is a joke. Various non-authoritative attempts at quality control are made, and one of them takes the form of the departmental "Morbidity and Mortality Conference" once every week or two. In these meetings mistakes and failures are aired, with the implied aim of improving doctor performance. Attendance is often lackadaisical, and the proceedings tepid and tentative. The doctors in the room know who the real culprits are, but the air is charged, the situation somewhat reminiscent of a gathering of bristling stray dogs circling and sniffing. Even the most accomplished specialist can't say too much. Some of his patients die, too. Unless this is a medical school hospital (or a renowned clinic) with a closed staff and a permanent chief of each specialty, there is no real authority in the room, because the meeting is run by doctors who themselves are involved in the same endeavors. This is not an effective way to bare accountability.

At these meetings in a teaching hospital, the resident presents the cases under study, and touchy questions are tentatively suggested. Blame hovers about, and the attending doctor rises to a display of forthrightness, in his largess accepting responsibility for an underling's actions, self-effacing yet defending himself and others by using the royal "we." Nothing else happens, and they go on to the next case, and next week. In some medical schools, the person in charge of a department, general surgery or urology, for instance, may be the least capable surgeon of his specialty in town. He may be all books and talk and political prominence in the academic circuit of his particular specialty, and no hands in the operating room. This irony destroys the myth of ultimate academic authority.

In either academic or town hospitals, there is no authority to which the behavior of individual doctors is accountable on a day-to-day and patient-to-patient basis except in the professionalism, the personal integrity, and the ability of each physician. No matter where the medical action may be, actually no one person or authority is in charge of the whole scene. Patients and their families should choose carefully and guard themselves and their friends even in the highest and mightiest accommodations.

News media sporadically accuse medical governing boards, at higher levels than the hospitals, of professional self-protection, and the exposé pushes for a stronger degree of legislated blame-placing. This approach only drives the doctors further underground. When they are being blamed for the failures in a system they do not control, they become defensive and are very careful about revealing damaging information.

Efforts now are being made outside of legislative regulation to apply the principles of corporate management to medicine. Mishaps would be regarded as system failures. The reporting of accidents would be encouraged, even rewarded, and no one would be persecuted for error, retrained perhaps, but not punished. This would remove the dangers to the doctors when they readily report errors regardless of who directly caused the problem. Without question the damaged patient deserves just compensation, and the entire system should develop a model to fill this need.

The system needs to be changed to prevent failures and to serve the patient's needs, and not for the convenience of the medical personnel handling patients in the hospital and office. This would end the current trend of depersonalizing patients for the sake of easier management. The change would arouse the patient and the patient's family to act with all the self-possession and authority used in other everyday endeavors.

Legislative quality control of conventional medicine, administered democratically, would entail the control of other healing endeavors as well, including faith healing, psychology, chiropractic, and all alternative medicine techniques. It won't be done for many years yet, but we can hope.

People in today's environment do not enter a hospital or a doctor's office to buy a commodity. The person as a patient goes for an occasion much like a trip where certain dangers are inherent in the under taking. just as anyone would look out for his own well-being and safety on a trek through the jungle, so he should do the same in the medical world, being his own or his relative's or his friend's guardian. Planes do crash and automobiles collide, always due to a human failure of one kind or another in the mechanics or in the operation. Accidents happen in medicine, too, and for the same reasons.

Your Choice

Decisions about treatment are crucial. Does the patient have a choice? Is there a better way? Will a person live longer if he leaves it alone and just does nothing? Is a surgical procedure an unnecessary and somewhat dangerous striving for perfection? Here are some examples:

A young man, 20 years old, in a line of recruits, received strong advice from a Navy doctor to have his varicocele (a varicose vein above a testicle) removed, with scary prognostications about loss of manhood, a big bag of veins dragging him down, fatal blood clots, and other terrible consequences if the operation were not done. He decided against the surgery. Sixty-four years later, at 84, and now the father of six children and the grandfather of 20, he is, with the help of a little pill, still making love twice a week, and the varicocele is no bigger.

A 75-year-old man had a benign tumor near the back of the brain on the nerve of hearing. The growth, doing no other harm, appeared big as a walnut on an MRI. The patient had survived two heart attacks, one triple bypass procedure, both femoral (thigh) arteries had been replaced with tubes of artificial material, and he was diabetic and nearly blind from retinopathy. The vascular disease would take him before the tumor could grow big enough to obstruct the fluid pathways of the brain. But it wasn't good enough for Daddy. The family ignored the advice to leave the tumor alone and found a surgeon in a world-renowned hospital and medical school. He downplayed the dangers, performed the operation, and three days later the family took Daddy home in a box.

Treatment can be worse than the disease. Total removal of a benign but difficult tumor by a daring surgeon can leave the area of the body laid waste like a battlefield. Fighting cancer with massive doses of radiation and chemotherapy can send the patient home with his body defenses ruined, exposing him to fatal infections. Will the prophylactic removal of both breasts really prevent cancer? Will the quality of life after treatment be nothing more than the brief extension of a miserable exodus? Will death be more painful after the treatment than it would have been without it? Would treatment of a brain tumor with the gamma knife or cyber knife (focused radiation) be as effective as a surgical procedure, without the risks? It's being tried now in several centers with encouraging results. Multiple benign tumors on both sides of the brain can be monitored over time by repeated MRI studies without treatment unless the tumors prove to be enlarging.

A patient is not bound to do what the doctor says. He does not belong to the doctor or owe him allegiance in any way, especially when it risks life or health. Should a patient be afraid of hurting the doctor's feelings? No, not if hesitancy might cost him dearly. Do fads in medicine threaten patients? Without doubt. For example, far too many hysterectomies and tonsillectomies were done in years past. The major surgical assaults on women with breast cancer are now no longer in vogue. Think carefully, investigate, and seek other opinions before accepting potentially dangerous, disfiguring, or unpleasant treatment.

Medicine, like any other body of knowledge, is open to any person capable of reading. One of the most remarkable privileges of modern life is the availability of information. No one can be kept ignorant if he learns to pursue knowledge readily available. Any time a disease, diagnosis, or treatment threatens, go to the Internet and tap into the wealth of medical writing available for everyone to use in solving health problems. Doctors can and do get it wrong for a number of reasons, and books and magazine articles written about the pitfalls in some of their thinking patterns evoke complicated psychological reasons for errors, and push psychology schemes to prevent errors. In fact, however, failures often can be blamed on the doctor's not following the simple basic principles of good practice. For instance, missing a classical case of aspirin poisoning simply means the doctor did not bother to take even a reasonably good history. Certainly every doctor needs to know what medicines his patient is taking and how much, what he is mixing with what, and what he is eating. Diagnostic medicine is detective work, and the answers come from many sources. Perhaps the most important of these is the patient himself. **Listen to the patient** is repeated to medical students from the beginning of their educations, but many doctors, in something of self defense, adopt instead the bad habits of impatience, the authoritative stance, the blindness of self-importance, the hurried put down interrupting the patient struggling with his words and the medical environment, and worst of all the pose of wisdom. Watch out for puffed-up old frauds trying to hide a lot of junk in their own screwed-up psyches. Any patient should raise his voice if his doctor is not listening.

HEALTH-CARE DELIVERY

The **term health-care delivery** is demeaning to the dignity of the ethical doctor of medicine, yet it comes pretty close to being an accurate description of how the system functions. What really drives it? What lies at the foot of medicine's immense progress in so few years after centuries of ignorance? The answer is, almost without exception, the laboratory. Most of the drugs in use today as well as modern diagnostic techniques from X-ray to the MRI are based on laboratory discoveries of modern times. Drugs and the entire gamut of chemicals used in medicine make it all possible. Without them, from anesthetics to antibiotics, surgery would be very limited. Live organ transplantation as we know it would never have happened. All life depends on complex body chemistry. All drugs, alternative medicine or otherwise, are chemicals, but all chemicals are not drugs. Drug companies spend large amounts of money on research in hopes of finding a miracle drug of enormous commercial value. This would be to the good of mankind's health, and even better for the drug company's coffers, and profits to the investors. Drug purchases help foot the bill for research.

Laboratories everywhere, including the rare climes of some ivory towers, go with the thrust of commercial enterprise. A university can be greatly enriched by the right patent on a revolutionary discovery. Capitalism at its best stimulates and inspires important progress, and has beneficial fallouts. Capitalism at its worst does not give a damn about the customer's health, except as it reflects on the sales of products. Drug companies want people to buy their concoctions as well as the pure drugs. Listen to their television ads about over-the-counter products and take their claims with critical doubt. Many times advertisements for prescription drugs end with the advice, "ask your doctor," then roll quickly through on the fine print at the bottom of the page too fast to be fully comprehended. Laws controlling drug advertising, weak as they are, require the revelation of certain adverse effects. The purpose of advertising is to sell, the purpose of selling is to make money, and advertising will play as close to misleading information as the law allows. These advertisements are using patients to put pressure on doctors to sell the advertised drugs. and try to turn every patient into a drug salesman of a sort. Also, and worse, the term "ask your doctor" carries another and even more malicious intent; it tries to shift the responsibility for drug damages on the doctor who cannot possibly know as much about a particular drug as should the drug manufacturer. In truth no one knows the ultimate effects of many drugs, even those in use for decades.

Aggressive marketing of Vioxx and Celebrex for the treatment of arthritis annually sold billions of dollars worth of the drugs before the cardiovascular complications were brought to light. The cardiologists who wrote the study and the publisher of the results were lobbied by the marketers of the drugs before results of this research were revealed (**Wall Street Journal**, August 22, 2001).

Yet, Vioxx was not taken off the market until late in the year 2004. Look at what happened with Fen-Phen, and all the hearts it damaged.

Supplies for the treatment and prevention of illness come from the manufacturers of drugs and medical devices, and the drugs and devices are delivered to patients through the doctors. There, with all the people who work to support the system, from pharmacists and nurses to aids and orderlies, is **health-care delivery**, a ridiculously overblown term with no real meaning. Doctors treat the ill and promote health by steering patients toward prevention and guiding them to sensible living and eating. And no one person can have all the facts. The answers have to be found in a morass of information and misinformation. For the sake of health and budget, dismiss most television advertisements as useless or misleading.

The doctor is caught up in the medical system of this nation. On the strength of his knowledge and expertise in the practice of medicine, he carries several major industries, three in particular: insurance, drugs, and hospitals. The drug companies depend on the doctor for delivery of all controlled drugs The hospital industry could not exist without the doctor. The patient's greatest expense does not come from the doctor; it comes from these three major industries. Through the lack of aggressive leadership in his profession, the doctor has become the servant of insurance. Insurance is there to make money for itself and for no other reason, and comprehensive medical insurance coverage is not available at any price. All policies are couched to protect the insurance companies, not the patient. But no one has been able to start and sustain a better system, and everybody fears government medicine. very likely it would entail a sluggish bureaucracy like the postal service or Social Security. The insurance problem has grown infinitely worse in recent years. Under the current circumstances, anyone who is not dirt poor on the one hand or very rich on the other is in real financial danger from potential medical disasters. What is left of the cottage industry in this country stands in the greatest danger. If such a small operator owns his own home or land or shop, small and humble as it is, he could be wiped out by one night in an emergency room. The medical system would strip him. This situation became worse during the Clinton administration when failed attempts to interfere with the system produced a financial vacuum in which only the large insurance carriers had the wherewithal to step in and take over. The concept of health maintenance organizations (HMO) dates back to the 1920s, and the early ones were non-profit plans, in other words, insurance against financial disaster. The profits were used to pay the costs and thus prevent the destructive debts. The well payers took care of the sicker payers. These plans were self-sustaining. Following the intervention of the federal government, this industry has come to exist for the primary purpose of making money for the investors. This trap needs to be removed and something like the initial HMO concept reinstated with improvements. The primary thrust of the hospital and the nursing home industries is profit; patient care lags behind (Cohn, J. *Sick:* Harper Collins 2007). Many of the current problems could be alleviated by a return to the original concept of an HMO.

The doctor has evolved over the ages since his appearance in the first semblance of tribal life. The doctor, priest, shaman, witchdoctor, medicine man, and the same people known under other names, were in the beginning both doctor and priest. Somewhere down the ages doctor and priest began to part ways, but only through a long and slow process, and the separation even today is not complete.

In the eyes of people struggling for a livelihood, the preacher and doctor are regarded as necessary evils to be tolerated, but never with full seriousness. The original tribal priest-medicine man had absolute power, but he had no means to rescue a patient other than ceremony. Magic and mystery gave him power in an atmosphere of superstition. Failures could be blamed on the patient's lack of real faith. Absolute power through mystery depends on the ignorance of the audience, usually also captive by circumstances. Down through the centuries, the medical doctor has been attacked for his failures and for his attitude. His critics have included William Shakespeare, Ben Jonson, and Moliere, along with many others. Conscientious formal training did him little good because he was then locked in by such conventions as blood letting. Only knowledge could and did free the doctors from these shackles. There are shackles to be broken yet.

As knowledge has grown for the patient, the power of mystery has diminished. The bonds of ignorance are being released by education. Yet the air of authority still works to empower the doctor and disarm the patient. Modern medicine is entirely autocratic, the product of dictatorial power structures, despotic in the higher levels. The medical hierarchy functions by put-downs to its members in descending order. Generalizations can be dangerous and not entirely accurate, but a chosen few, not necessarily the smarter or more ambitious doctors, tend to stay around the medical schools and renowned clinics after completing a course of training. Those in higher places rule by disdain. In the present system they train the best they can get. These and others who are less fortunate men are used as cheap labor while in training, and then they go out on the public without any real control of their professional behavior afterward. Once outside the academic setting, these people do more or less as they please—or what is worse, more or less as they can—for the rest of their careers. They are accountable to no real restraint other than their own conscience, and perhaps, ultimately, a plaintiff's attorney. Some are first rate; others are far less.

These same autocrats control the specialty boards, specialty training programs, editorial boards of the medical journals, the politics of the medical societies, and liaison with government. They also control continued education in the form of national meetings, and re-examinations, the latter actually a disguised method of retaining political power for themselves. Certifying boards take no responsibility for the quality of the performance of doctors who have passed the examinations, and their spokesmen say certification does not imply competence; they say so and they pay a host of lawyers to protect them in this stance.

The fatal flaw of medicine is the lack of effective organization and leadership. Usually, the highest ambition of the medical politician is to become president of his particular medical society, from the lowest to the highest, from the smallest to the largest, a post lasting only one year. This system never chooses anyone truly qualified to lead medicine where it needs to go in the twenty-first century. The big event for any medical society no matter how big or how small in the entire USA is the annual, local, state, or national meeting, a convention more a combination of circus and country fair than scientific and educational. The show is for the people putting it on, where they are seen in power, but it is also where they meet to control the politics and entertain a chosen few with cocktails and special banquets at the expense of the entire membership, while the IRS sleeps. The majority members and attendees are held at bay, perhaps in awe, by the pomp and ceremony.

In recent years, the leadership of some surgical groups has taken to inviting past presidents of the United States, noted journalists the likes of George Will and Thomas L. Friedman, movie moguls such as George Lucas, and other notables from society at large to speak at the plenary sessions, perhaps in the hopes of real importance rubbing off. The annual banquet, for all members who pay the extra fee, is a stage for displaying the grandeur of the current president and his inevitably wonderful wife, whose abidance and tolerance made his extraordinary accomplishments possible. Such statements as, "I couldn't have done it without her," and "I'm honored to be your president," are heard on this occasion every year. Past presidents come up to the podium and open packages and give out little gifts and put ribbons around necks. The entire scene carries the air of an insider joke and calls for a cessation of intelligence in the audience subjected to this empty exercise. No thinking person who attends one of these meetings to keep up with progress comes away thinking well of himself or his specialty.

This same limp leadership exists at every level of organized medicine from the meekest county society to the largest national societies, and all the specialty organizations in the United States. Until medicine becomes organized under effective leadership, it will continue on its present damaged path. Only in such strength can it regain control of its own destiny and resist the overpowering insurance industry, the corporate hospital systems, and the drug companies. Only in such strength can it control the faults of its own members. Organized medicine must learn to discipline its own ranks and to remedy other faults responsible for the present unwieldy and unhappy situation.

Here is a quotation from the first code of ethics of the American Medical Association, 1847: "Physicians … should unite tenderness with firmness and condescension with authority... The obedience of a patient ... should be prompt and implicit ... (the patient) should never permit his own crude opinions as to their fitness."

In the twenty-first century, medicine can no longer use this arrogant bluff. Imagine the ignorance being hidden and defended more than 150 years ago behind such puffery. Those were the days before the discovery of germs, and anesthesia was just being born (1844-1847: Wells and Morton; see the Internet for numerous references). Fortunately for the patient, this attitude today protects the system much less as the information age grows. Knowledge of medicine no longer belongs to the doctor's domain alone. As the public becomes more informed, medicine has to assume a growing responsibility for its actions. It is the patient who should be and is becoming empowered.

On the scene of sudden and grave illness or injury, patients and their families quickly find themselves in a passive role. Illness weakens the patient and renders him dependent, and the families, frightened by the circumstances and the proceedings, try to cooperate and not interfere. The scene can be awesome, the patient helpless, a life in other hands, tubes and lines from every direction, nurses bent over the victim administering mercy angels in white, doctors in operating clothes, the only and the last authority between man and god. There can be no sweeter or more humbling picture, and every reasonable human being appreciates its significance and honors its rights. This authority serves its purpose well in a dire emergency, but when protracted full time, the world of medicine cannot live up to the responsibility because it is run by people, and regardless of the endeavor, people are more or less the same universally. Any fault or mishap in one arena of human activity will occur in the others, but the privileges granted to medicine by society create an extraordinary leeway for both error and deliberate misconduct. These faults only become worse when no one challengers the activities. Therein lies a major source of trouble. No one can afford to assign responsibility for his own safety entirely to a system of any kind, whether in the medical jungle, or the tropical jungle, or on the Interstate, or on a boating party, or wherever.

Despite its faults, the medical system in the Western world saves thousands of lives every day, often with knowledge and techniques only dreamed of a generation past. It would be foolhardy to stay away altogether because of the faults. Most of its errors fall under the category of stupid mistakes. These can be avoided with a little thought and painstaking attention to detail, and by adherence to a system of double-checking everything risky. Most doctors are good men and women who want patients to get well without problems of any kind. But in self-defense people must always be aware of the particular circumstances of the medical system. As with the jungle, people go to it; it does not come to them, and unprepared or unwary, they go there on its terms.

WEB SITES

Bloodbook: Information for Life
www.bloodbook.com

ClinicalTrials: A Service of the National Institutes of Health
www.clinicaltrials.gov

HealthGrades
www.healthgrades.com

Joint Commission on Accreditation of Healthcare Organizations
www.jcaho.org

Legalzoom online legal services
www.legalzoom.com

MedicAlert
www.medicalert.org

The National Consumers League
www.nclnet.org

The Physician's Desk Reference
www.pdr.net.

The Skeptic's Dictionary
www.skepdic.com

BIBLIOGRAPHY

Angell, Marcia, M.D. **The Truth about the Drug Companies: How They Deceive Us and What to Do about It** (NY: Random House, 2004)

Avorn, Jerry, M.D. **Powerful Medicines: The Benefits, Risks, and Costs of Prescription Drugs** (NY: Knopf, 2004)

Berg, MB, Tymoczko, JL, and Stryer, LS, **Biochemistry** (NY: W.H. Freeman and Company)

Carroll, Robert Todd. **The Skeptic's Dictionary: A Collection of Strange Beliefs, Amusing Deceptions, and Dangerous Delusions** (NY: John Wiley & Sons, 2003)

Changuex, J-P, Riceour, P. **What Makes Us Think?** (NY: Princeton University Press, 2000)

Cohn, J. **Sick** (Harper Collins, 2007)

Coveney, P. and Highfield, R. **Frontiers of Complexity: The Search for Order in a Chaotic World** (New York: Fawcett Columbine, 1995)

Ernst, Edzard. "A primer of complimentary and alternative medicine commonly used by cancer patients." (**www.mja.com.au/publiclissues/174_02_150101/lernst/ernst.html**)

Guyton, Arthur C., and John E. Hall. **Textbook of Medical Physiology, Ninth Edition** (Philadelphia, PA: W B Saunders Co, 1996)

Hardman, Joel G., and Lee E. Limbird, editors. **Goodman and Gilman's The Pharmacological Basis of Therapeutics, Tenth Edition** (NY: McGraw-Hill, 2001)

Margolis, Simeon. **The Johns Hopkins Consumer Guide to Drugs** (NY: Rebus, 2002)

PDR staff. **Physician's Desk Reference, 59th Edition 2005**

Wootton, David. **BAD MEDICINE** (Oxford University Press, 2006)

Made in the USA
San Bernardino, CA
28 September 2016